Child Language

Multilingual Matters

The Age Factor in Second Language Acquistion
  D. SINGLETON and Z. LENGYEL (eds)
Building Bridges
  MULTILINGUAL RESOURCES FOR CHILDREN PROJECT
Competing and Consensual Voices
  PATRICK J.M. COSTELLO and SALLY MITCHELL (eds)
Foundations of Bilingual Education and Bilingualism
  COLIN BAKER
Language, Minority Education and Gender
  DAVID CORSON
Language Reclamation
  HUBISI NWENMELY
Multicultural Child Care
  P. VEDDER, E. BOUWER and T. PELS
A Parents' and Teachers' Guide to Bilingualism
  COLIN BAKER
Researching the Early Years Continuum
  PAT BROADHEAD (ed.)
The Step-Tongue: Children's English in Singapore
  ANTHEA FRASER GUPTA
Three Generations – Two Languages – One Family
  LI WEI
The World in a Classroom
  V. EDWARDS and A. REDFERN
Working with Bilingual Children
  M.K. VERMA, K.P. CORRIGAN and S. FIRTH (eds)

Please contact us for the latest book information:
Multilingual Matters Ltd, Frankfurt Lodge, Clevedon Hall,
Victoria Road, Clevedon, Avon, England, BS21 7SJ.

Child Language

Edited by
Michelle Aldridge

MULTILINGUAL MATTERS LTD
Clevedon • Philadelphia • Adelaide

Library of Congress Cataloging in Publication Data

Child Language
Edited by Michelle Aldridge
1. Children–Language–Congresses. 2. Language aquisition–Congresses.
3. Language disorders in children–Congresses. 4. Linguistics–Congresses.
5. Bilingualism in children–Congresses.
I. Aldridge, Michelle. II. Child Language Seminar (1994: University of Wales)
LB1139.L3C4366   1994
401.93–dc20   95-23852

British Library Cataloguing in Publication Data

A CIP catalogue record for this book is available from the British Library.

ISBN 1-85359-316-8 (hbk)

Multilingual Matters Ltd

UK: Frankfurt Lodge, Clevedon Hall, Victoria Road, Clevedon, Avon BS21 7SJ.
USA: 1900 Frost Road, Suite 101, Bristol, PA 19007, USA.
Australia: P.O. Box 6025, 83 Gilles Street, Adelaide, SA 5000, Australia.

Typeset by Formatvisual, Weston-super-Mare.
Printed and bound in Great Britain by WBC Book Manufacturers Ltd.

Contents

Introduction

The Child Language Seminar is an annual event. Each year a different British University provides the venue for this occasion and in the Spring of 1994 I had the good fortune to host this three day conference here in North Wales. Thus, on the lunchtime of Monday March 28th, 87 delegates began to register for what would hopefully be three days of lively debate from 31 oral paper presentations and nine poster displays. We were also joined by Blackwell, Cambridge, Langlearn Communications, Paramount and Whurr publishers.

The conference was opened by the subjects themselves. Six children under five years of age from our University Nursery Tir na n-Og (Celtic for 'Land of the young') came to one of the lecture halls and sang a 'welcome song' in Welsh and English. From that point onwards we knew that we were going to have an enjoyable as well as beneficial time together.

The proceedings here represent most of the papers and to those I'll return in a while. I would first, however, like to reflect on our guest speakers. We were privileged to have five.

On the Monday evening at a wine reception *Professor Tim Miles, University of Wales, Bangor* gave a fascinating talk entitled *Developmental Dyslexia: An unusual balance of skills.* He overviewed his long and established career in dyslexia focusing on causes, symptoms as well as remedial strategies. On Tuesday evening, *Professor Nina Hyams, University of California* addressed the issue of *The underspecification of functional categories.* This was a state-of-the art presentation of the status of children's earliest grammatical clauses in keeping with the continuity theory of language acquisition. On Wednesday morning, *Professors Harald Clahsen and Andrew Radford, University of Essex* continued the theme of syntactic development with their paper *Clause structure in early child language acquisition* and gave further arguments in this controversial area of language development from slightly different perspectives from that of Nina. Andrew's paper is included here. Our other guest speaker was *Professor David Crystal, professor emeritus from the University of Wales, Bangor* who gave a wonderful after-dinner speech, following the conference dinner on Tuesday evening, entitled *Child language: the greatest story never told.* Here he mixed serious academic points, with childhood humour and anecdotal stories to the extent that everyone in the room ached with laughter but also through sheer admiration of his ability to illustrate our interactions with children and the mistakes *we* make. There wasn't a dry eye in the hall – through pleasure of course.

CLS aims to further our understanding of all aspects of child development and to this end delegates were welcomed from all disciplines. The time was shared with academics, child psychologists, pediatricians, speech therapists and teachers. Topics thus fell into broad categories such as bilingualism, exceptional language and literacy, linguistic theory, language disorders, pre-linguistic development and signed languages.

The proceedings offer a flavour of the conference. All contributors were invited to submit their oral or poster presentation to this volume. In total 17 of the possible 40 presentations are offered here. Summarising the conference, on Monday, we had a single session focusing on the acquisition of phonology. The paper here from *Reid et al.* represents this session. On Tuesday we had parallel sessions all day, with Session A focusing on non-syntactic development. Papers here from *Clibbens et al., Franco et al., Gallaway et al.* and *Wait* are typical of Session A while Session B focused on syntactic development with contributions such as *Hamann, Koster et al.* and *Yamada-Yamamoto.* Wednesday morning saw us focusing on grammatical language impairment with papers such as *King* and *Van der Lely* and on the modelling of language acquisition with presentations from *Abidi et al., Fowler et al.,* and *Taylor.*

Delegates came from America, Canada, England, Finland, Germany, Holland, Scotland, Spain, Switzerland, and Wales. We shared different experiences and research knowledge and came away with renewed friendship and determination to further our understanding of child development. CLS 1995 will be held in Bristol. I wish them every success in their preparation and look forward to seeing some old friends and colleagues there. Thank you to everyone who made CLS 1994 such a pleasurable experience including, of course, my two helpers *Samantha Bedwell* and *Alun Waddon.* The following captures most of the papers and posters presented at Bangor.

Michelle Aldridge

1 Child Language Development: A Connectionist Simulation of the Evolving Concept Memory

SYED SIBTE RAZA ABIDI AND KHURSHID AHMAD

Connectionist networks, *or the so-called* neural networks, *provide a basis for studying child language development, in that these networks emphasise learning, either from observations or from being told, and that the design of these networks simplifies questions related to the representation of linguistic and world knowledge through the use of a network of 'simple' nodes and links. We report a connectionist simulation of child language development, essentially focusing on the development of children's concepts. We demonstrate how a connectionist network can learn concepts in an unsupervised manner; exhibiting evidence of an 'indirect' learning of categories leading to the emergence of a category structure. The data used in the simulation have their origins in the longitudinal psycholinguistic study of children through their various stages of cognitive development, including sensori-motor and pre-operational stages. The concept representation scheme for simulating a child's concept memory is semantic feature-oriented (Nelson, 1973) and the concepts learnt are taken from the archives of Lois Bloom (1973). The connectionist simulation was carried out using ACCLAIM — A* Connectionist Child LAnguage development and Imitation Model. *ACCLAIM is a modular connectionist architecture comprising 'supervised' and 'unsupervised' learning connectionist networks, and takes into account the diverse nature of inputs to and outputs from a child learning his or her first language.*

Introduction

Learning is a much debated topic in artificial intelligence (AI), neurobiology and linguistics. The studies in child language development are at once an exemplar of and an inspiration to workers in human learning. Child language has a body of systematically collected data, and is an aspect of human development that has, thus far, eluded a well-grounded, objective theoretical framework. We believe that the study of child language development can benefit from the objectivity that may be implicit in connectionist network methodology.

Child language development theories have motivated the collection of substantial amounts of observational data. The data collection exercises involve a number of interesting hypotheses about how a child may perceive the 'world' around himself or herself. This may include his or her beliefs, desires and feelings. In order to express such internal states, Bloom has argued that language development needs to account for the development of concepts, lexica, semantics, syntax and discourse (1993:96). Therefore, it is possible to argue that if one were successful in synthesising psycholinguistic observations, particularly during the various stages of language development, spanning the onset of language (c. 9–12 months), the vocabulary spurt, and the transition to multi-word speech (c. 18–24 months), with the developmental neurobiological observations, then one might have a psychologically plausible and neurobiologically tangible description of the language of children.

Advances in neurobiology have inspired computing scientists to build systems that crudely mimic the organisation of the brain; the so-called neural networks or connectionist networks are potentially parallel processing systems, involving co-operative computations among locally connected processing units. Their crudity notwithstanding, and the fact that much of what inspired the early neural network pioneers were simplistic notions in behaviourism, neural networks have one important characteristic that makes them more plausible than, say, artificially intelligent systems or conventional procedural computing systems. This characteristic is their ability to 'learn' from observations and from stimuli over a period of time; learning is inherent in the design of connectionist networks, whereas both the conventional and AI systems are incapable of such learning. Bechtel and Abrahamsen have argued that 'connectionism could be viewed as a modern mechanism for achieving stage-like states by means of the heretofore somewhat mysterious processes of accommodation and assimilation' (1991:271).

Simulations of problem-solving behaviour in artificial intelligence, though not overtly mathematical while remaining algorithmic, have led to a better understanding of problem-solving behaviour. The same could perhaps be said about developments in computational linguistics, particularly the development of programs that syntactically analyse phrases and sentences. The success of simulation-based studies in physics, chemistry and biology, and more recently in computational linguistics, has inspired a number of workers including Siskind (1990), MacWhinney (1987), Hill (1983), Langley (1982) and Selfridge (1986) to build simulation models of child language development. These studies were either based on methods and techniques used in conventional computer science or in artificial intelligence.

Such simulations, though very instructive, cannot be used to explicate much about learning, insofar as the conventional computing and AI systems used in child language simulation studies do not have any learning mechanisms. In any case, the focus of these studies was on procedural aspects of human problem-solving. Connectionist simulation appears more promising in the context of child language development, through its underpinnings in neurobiology and psychology, while the learning mechanisms inherent in the design of connectionist networks might allow a better simulation of child language development.

Our own work is different from the earlier simulations of child language development in three significant respects: first, we simulate a number of aspects of human language including lexical organisation and access, conceptual memory, semantics, pivot grammar and word order for studying evolving linguistic behaviour. Second, our focus is on the *development* or the evolution of linguistic behaviour amongst children. The notions of innate structures notwithstanding, language is learnt over a period of time and involves environmental input. This includes input from the physical environment, caretakers, siblings and others, together with language learnt by the child on his or her own initiative with or without supervision, either through the maturity of the nervous system or through some other natural gift. Third, we believe that the interdependence of language learnt via environmental input and self-motivated language learning can surely influence the kinds of connectionist network architectures that either simulate 'supervised learning' or 'unsupervised learning'.

We have developed ACCLAIM — A Connectionist Child LAnguage development and Imitation Model to simulate child language development within the age group 9–24 months. ACCLAIM is a modular connectionist architecture implementing a variety of connectionist networks, including *Kohonen maps, backpropagation networks, additive Grossberg networks,* and networks with *Hebbian connections* incorporating the *spreading activation* mechanism. ACCLAIM has been used to simulate the development of concepts in children together with the lexicalisation of these concepts: the *concept memory* and *word lexicon* have been simulated using Kohonen maps and are linked together through a Hebbian connection-based *concept lexicalisation* network. Backpropagation networks have been used to implement a *conceptual relation* network (for one-word sentences) and a *word-order* network (for two-word sentences). Children's evolving 'semantic' performance has been simulated using an additive Grossberg network. Thus, aspects of what can be construed to be innate development have been simulated using networks with unsupervised learning regimes, such as Kohonen maps and Hebbian connections, and environmentally-determined features of language development have been simulated using networks with supervised learning regimes, such as backpropagation networks. ACCLAIM has been trained on 'realistic' child language data and has learnt to recognise and produce one-word and two-word sentences.

Connectionism: A Brief Introduction

Connectionism is a research discipline that aims to understand the nature of human intelligence by simulating aspects of human behaviour through a collection of idealised neurons. Connectionism draws much of its inspiration from neuroscience in that the *neuron* is taken as the basic *processing unit*. Each processing unit is characterised by an *activation level* (analogous to the state of polarisation of a neuron), an *output value* (representing the firing rate of the neuron), and a set of *input* and *output connections* (representing the neuron's dendrites and axons) to and from other units, respectively. These characteristics are expressed in a mathematical formalism such that a unit's activation level and output value are expressed as (real) numbers, and its connections with other units have an associated *weight* (synaptic strength) which determines the effect of the incoming input on the activation level of the unit. The processing units are provided with a variety of 'stimuli' and are expected to 'respond' in a manner that mimics aspects of human behaviour.

Learning in a connectionist network

Learning in connectionist networks is deeply rooted in the work of behavioural psychologists during the 1940s and 1950s. Textbooks on connectionist networks begin with statements such as 'learning would involve relatively enduring changes in a system of given architecture that results from its interaction with the environment. The most obvious form of learning is adjustment in the weights of connections' (Bechtel & Abrahamsen, 1991:270).

Learning is effected through changes in the strength of connections between individual processing units in a connectionist network. Put simply, given a set of inputs $x_1, x_2, \ldots x_n$ (a vector symbolically denoted as X) to a system, the system generates a set of outputs, $y_1, y_2, \ldots y_m$ denoted symbolically as (a vector) Y. This is achieved computationally by relating X and Y through a matrix of connection weights denoted as W:

$$W = \left[\begin{pmatrix} w_{11} & w_{12} & ... & w_{1n} \\ w_{21} & w_{22} & ... & w_{2n} \\ . & . & & . \\ . & . & & . \\ . & . & & . \\ w_{m1} & w_{m2} & ... & w_{mn} \end{pmatrix} \right]$$

This interrelationship matrix assumes that one, some or all the inputs influence individual outputs: $y_m = w_{m1}x_1 + w_{m2}x_2 + ... + w_{mn}x_n$. Learning in the above simplification is then the change of the weights, ΔW.

Some connectionists and philosophers of science have reinterpreted Piagetian notions of learning in the connectionist paradigm. Specifically, this reinterpretation focuses on the Piagetian notions of *accommodation* and *assimilation*. For instance, McClelland's essay on the implications of connectionism for 'cognition and development' includes the description of a 'learning principle' governing cognitive development: 'adjust the parameters of the mind in proportion to the extent to which their adjustment can produce a reduction in the discrepancy between expected and observed events' (1989:20).

ACCLAIM — A Connectionist Child Language Development and Imitation Model

Consider the following model of child language development: (i) the child receives two types of input from his or her environment: one is perceptual input that enables the child to categorise entities and events, and the other is linguistic input in the form of the caretaker's language, mainly as 'two-word collocates'; (ii) the innate ability of the brain then helps the child to understand his or her environment, abstracting critical semantic features to form concepts and storing them in a *concept memory*; (iii) the child also discriminates between the phonetic content of the linguistic input from caretakers to develop a repertoire of words — the word lexicon; (iv) at the end of sensori-motor development, the child learns functional words or 'conceptual relations', and learns to use them as single-word utterances, each in different situations that have common contexts; (v) the child learns to associate concepts and words in an unsupervised manner; (vi) the child generalises further and creates the so-called conceptual categories leading to the development of 'semantic relations' among conceptual categories; (vii) finally, the child, through a process of trial and error, builds up collocates that conform to the word order in his or her caretaker's language, leading to the production of child-like two-word sentences.

The above-mentioned aspects of the model (i–vii) can be simulated by individual connectionist networks or 'connectionist modules'. Some of these processes can be simulated by the so-called connectionist supervised learning algorithms whilst others can be simulated by the use of unsupervised learning algorithms. Unsupervised connectionist networks learn on their own without any explicit supervision — a type of learning which is seemingly more akin to some aspects of learning observed in a developing child.

A connectionist system that contains a number of (differing) networks, each performing a task in a plausible manner, can be referred to as a modular connectionist architecture. ACCLAIM was developed by organising independent connectionist networks in a psycholinguistically plausible manner. Figure 1.1 shows the modular architecture of ACCLAIM.

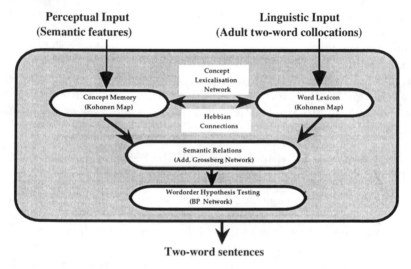

Figure 1.1 The modular connectionist architecture of ACCLAIM

In ACCLAIM all the simulations are carried out in a 'developmental' manner. Starting with no *a priori* information, the connectionist networks are exposed to a set of input stimuli — the so-called training patterns. Over a period of time (iterations), the connectionist networks are trained using the input stimuli, and at the end of the training, learn to recognise or to respond to the stimuli. Environmental influence during learning is demonstrated by the adaptability of the 'plastic' structure of the connectionist networks to account for information received from the environment.

Children's Conceptual Development: A Representation Scheme for a Connectionist Simulation

In order to represent concepts in a connectionist environment, we have adopted a conventional 'semantic feature' based formalism which describes the similarities and differences between various concepts and also helps in defining categories. Each concept in our connectionist representation scheme is represented by a 20-dimensional semantic feature vector comprising two types of features: 'defining features' — determining a category structure, and 'individual features' — distinguishing individual concepts within a category. We discuss below how these defining and individual features are used to construct a semantic feature vector for representing a concept.

The defining features of concepts in our simulation are based on an 'object-oriented' taxonomy — a hierarchical tree distinguishing features at each level. This particular taxonomy was suggested by Nelson (1973). For representing various objects and non-objects a child might encounter, we have labelled Nelson's hierarchical structures in terms of binary digits (1 and 0). Two categories at the same level of the tree, for instance 'objects' and 'non-objects', are assigned the values 1 and 0, respectively. Similarly, for the category 'object', the sub-category 'animate' is assigned the value 1 and 'inanimate' is assigned the value 0. Once the tree is labelled (see Figure 1.2), one can ascertain the 'defining features' for a concept by using the value '1' to indicate that the object/non-object contains a particular feature and '0' to indicate otherwise. Therefore, according to this representation scheme, concepts belonging to the *objects(1)–animate(1)–animal(0)–general(0)* category, for instance 'dog', are labelled [1 1 0 0].

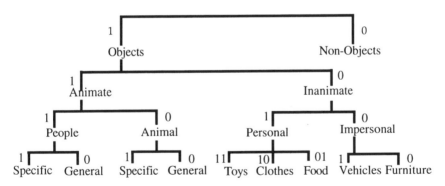

Figure 1.2 A cross-section of Nelson's semantic structure. Each branch is labelled with a binary value

In our representation scheme, the individual features are based on a taxonomy of children's concepts suggested by Bloom (1973) and recently commented upon by Anisfeld (1984). The taxonomy consists of seven different categories: *objects, agents, events, states, locations, prepositions,* and *function words* (expressing personal intentions, commands and desires). Each category comprises a number of 'individual features' that we believe may represent the concepts associated with the category. In Figure 1.3, we show a cross-section of the individual feature tree for the category *agents*, mainly focusing on features related to *human beings*. The individual features of a particular concept, for instance 'Dad', can be obtained by translating the constituent individual features into binary digits:

Agents → Human → Human Beings → Not self → Familiar → Does care → Is Kin →Male → Size (Large) → Has Name → 'Dad'

Individual features for 'Dad'   =   [1, 1, 0, 0, 1, 1, 1, 1, 1, 1]

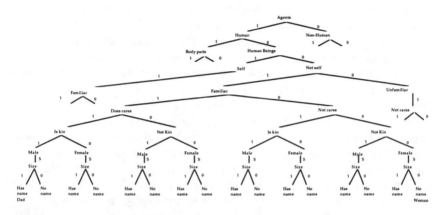

Figure 1.3 A cross-section of the individual feature tree for the category 'agents'. This figure shows the individual features for concepts identifying 'human beings'

Simulation of the Development of the 'Concept Memory'

We believe that one can model children's concepts, comprising objects, people, places and events through representation and categorisation in terms of a number of 'semantic features'. The learning of new concepts can, to a certain extent, be regarded as an unsupervised process, whereby children appear to detect the salient semantic features of a concept without any guidance.

We have simulated a concept memory comprising 43 'concepts'. This was achieved by using a 121 unit Kohonen map, which uses an unsupervised learning regime. The 43 concepts were selected from the range of concepts reported in child language literature (Bloom, 1973); each concept is represented by a 20-dimensional semantic feature vector.

The 43 concepts were initially presented to the 121 unit matrix designated to be the conceptual memory. Each concept was randomly assigned to one of the units in the conceptual memory (see Figure 1.4 page 11). Kohonen's unsupervised learning algorithm helps in the identification or construction of a small number of key 'features' of a given pattern or a cognitive task. This algorithm results in the creation of a spatially-organised feature map based on the adaptive units of the network. Feature detectors gradually develop such that given an input stimuli, the location of the excited units becomes indicative of the key features of the input. Given a set of input patterns (the so-called environment of the connectionist network), learning in unsupervised connectionist networks is accomplished by discovering statistical regularities in the input data. This involves the computation of a distance measure between the various concepts, based on the difference between the vectors representing each of the concepts.

The simulation of the development of the concept memory was carried out in an iterative manner, such that in each iteration a different concept was presented to the concept memory. The repeated presentation of the concepts over a number of iterations may be analogous to the child's increased appreciation and knowledge of the concept over a period of time. For the child, it is perhaps this frequent repetition of information which leads to its assimilation. Individual concepts were presented more than once in a random order to ensure that the 'learning' taking place was not biased in any way and did not reflect a predefined course of development.

To learn the concepts, the various output units *compete* to represent the input pattern, such that the unit acquiring the highest activation level *wins* the competition and is deemed to represent that particular input pattern. The weight vectors of the winning unit and its neighbouring units are then modified in alignment with the input pattern. Given that the concepts are learnt, i.e. represented by individual units in the Kohonen map, learning can be quantified in terms of two parameters — (i) the activation level (ACT) of the desired concept's unit when retrieved and (ii) the 'Euclidean distance' (ED) between the desired concept's unit and the most highly active unit. A concept is deemed to be learnt when, upon presentation of its semantic feature vector, the activation level of its representative unit is the highest amongst all other units (approaching unity), and its ED is the lowest (closest to zero). Learning a concept ensures that it is retrieved when its corresponding semantic feature vector is presented to the concept memory.

By way of describing this complex simulation, we discuss the learning profile of just one concept, 'dog' out of the 43 concepts to be learnt. Starting the simulation with a random Kohonen map (shown in Figure 1.4, page 11), the network was presented the 20-dimensional feature vector of each of the 43 concepts in a random order, during a learning period spanning 8000 iterations. To check how the Kohonen map learnt over the 8000 iterations, we interrupted the training at intervals of 500 iterations and took a snapshot of the evolving concept memory. For each snapshot we presented to the Kohonen map the semantic feature vector for the concept 'dog'. This resulted in all the Kohonen map units acquiring some activation level. The unit with the highest activation level was regarded as the concept retrieved. Table 1.1 gives a learning profile comprising the concept unit retrieved, and the activation level (ACT) and Euclidean distance (ED) of the concept unit 'dog'.

Table 1.1 Iteration-by-iteration learning of the concept 'dog'

Iteration		Stimulus = 'DOG'	
Range	Retrieved Unit	ACT	ED
1–500	pig	−0.27	0.335
501–1000	dog	−0.29	0.372
1000–1500	duck	0.170	0.366
1501–2000	duck	−0.29	0.096
2001–2500	dog	0.45	0.247
2501–3000	dog	0.966	0.003
3001–3500	dog	0.998	0.001
3501–4000	dog	1.0	0.0
4001–4500	dog	1.0	0.0
4501–5000	dog	1.0	0.0
5001–5500	dog	1.0	0.0
5501–6000	dog	1.0	0.0
6001–8000	dog	1.0	0.0

From the very first iteration, the ED between the weight vector of all the units and the input stimulus is computed. The unit that has the minimal distance to the stimulus is 'assigned' the stimulus label. Subsequent iterations involve the computation of the ED and the reassigning of concepts to the units. After the first 500 iterations, when the stimulus 'dog' is presented to the concept memory, the Kohonen map retrieves the concept 'pig' — that is, the Kohonen map has not yet learnt to discriminate between a 'dog' and a 'pig' and can easily confuse the two. This 'confused' behaviour of the Kohonen map can be explained as follows: the semantic feature representations of both concepts — 'pig' and 'dog' share a number of features. The retrieval of the proximate concept 'pig' instead of the concept 'dog' clearly indicates that, at this stage, the Kohonen map has acquired an understanding of a category structure, i.e. the defining features have been learnt. However, the Kohonen map is still not able to discriminate among the individual features of the concepts 'dog' and 'pig' (both concepts belong to the same category) and therefore confuses the stimulus 'dog' with the close concept 'pig'.

At the end of 1000 iterations, the stimulus 'dog' retrieves the unit labelled 'dog', but the value of the ED is quite large (0.372) and the activation level is very low — in fact it is negative (−0.29). This retrieval may yet turn out to be merely coincidental. This is confirmed at the end of

1500 and 2000 iterations: the Kohonen map now confuses the concept 'dog' with 'duck'. But after 2500 iterations, we see a positive activation and a reduction of the ED in the learning profile for the concept 'dog'. Subsequent iterations do show that the network is becoming more 'stable' in its response to the stimulus 'dog': a doubling of the activation level between 2500 and 4000 iterations and more than a 200 fold reduction in the ED. At iteration 4000, the criteria for adequate learning have been satisfied, i.e. the activation level has approached unity and the ED has decreased to zero. Figure 1.5 shows the organisation of the concept memory after a learning session of 8000 iterations, where each concept is represented by a unique unit.

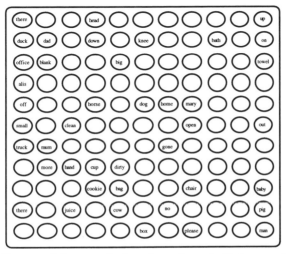

Figure 1.4 Concept Memory before learning: A Kohonen feature map without any training.

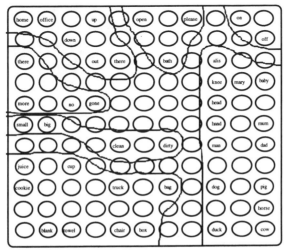

Figure 1.5 Concept Memory after learning: A Kohonen feature map after training (8000 iterations).

An indirect simulation of category learning: Evidence of a category structure

The organisation of the concept memory (as shown in Figure 1.5) at the end of the simulation shows evidence of a category structure (shown by solid lines). If one believes that categories are a means of making sense of the environment, then one can argue that although during the simulation there was no direct emphasis on category learning, the connectionist network, on its own 'initiative' (unsupervised learning), succeeded in learning certain categories.

Recognition of new concepts by a 'learnt' concept memory

The categorisation of learnt concepts helps in the recognition of new concepts, through the comparison of the features of concepts in existing categories with the features of the new concepts. For instance, a child may identify a new concept 'cat' in terms of a known and similar concept 'dog' because the new concept 'cat' has features that the child perceives are in common with the concept 'dog', e.g. 'has a tail', 'has a furry coat', 'roams in the house', 'is a pet' and so on.

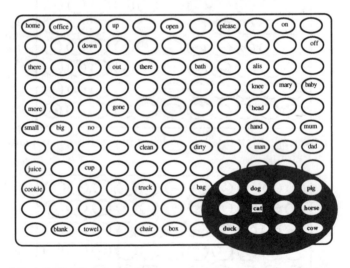

Figure 1.6 ACCLAIM recognises a concept 'cat', with which it was not familiar by virtue of its training, and categorises it correctly by placing 'cat' amongst other 'animals' the network was trained on.

We demonstrate the pattern recognition capability of the trained Kohonen map (Fig. 1.6). The map was presented with the feature vector describing a cat. This stimulus resulted in the feature map being temporarily modified to the extent that 'cat' now appears in the map, placed correctly amongst agents and specifically amongst animals. However, if a new concept were to be learnt, then the Kohonen feature map would need to be retrained with the previous concepts, in addition to the new concept.

Conclusion

We have presented a concept representation scheme based on 'defining' and 'individual' features. We have attempted to demonstrate that connectionist networks provide a basis for simulating concept development and for investigating human category learning. Our simulation of concept development displayed category learning effects and showed how unsupervised learning algorithms can be gainfully used for simulation. This is different from supervised learning, which mainly involves attaching category labels. We have attempted to show that the behaviour of self-organising connectionist networks may have some parallel with human learning, and that the design of such connectionist networks simplifies questions related to the representation of world knowledge through the use of simple nodes and links.

The emergence of connectionist network architectures — structures with a propensity for learning through instruction and experience — provides substantial opportunities for operationalising child language data and for testing theories relating to child language development. Using ACCLAIM, a number of other connectionist simulations have been carried out. They relate to naming development, to the development of the word lexicon, to the understanding of semantic relationships between words and between concepts, and finally to word-order development. These will further reinforce the above conclusion (Abidi, 1994).

Acknowledgements

One of the authors (SSRA) wishes to acknowledge a grant from Ministry of Science and Technology, Government of Pakistan towards supporting work on his doctoral dissertation.

References

Abidi, S.S.R. (1994) A connectionist simulation of child language development. Unpublished doctoral thesis, Department of Mathematical and Computing Sciences, University of Surrey, Guildford, UK.

Anisfeld, M. (1984) *Language Development From Birth to Three*. Hove and Hillsdale, NJ: Lawrence Erlbaum Associates.

Bechtel, W. and Abrahamsen, A. (1991) *Connectionism and the Mind*. Oxford: Basil Blackwell.

Bloom, L. (1973) *One Word at a Time*. Paris: Mouton.

— (1993) Language acquisition and the power of expression. In H. Roitblat, L. Herman and P. Nachtigall (eds) *Language and Communication*. Hillsdale, NJ: Lawrence Erlbaum Associates.

Hill, J. (1983) A computational model of language acquisition in the two-year-old. *Cognition and Brain Theory* 6, 287–317.

Langley, P. (1982) Language acquisition through error recovery. *Cognition and Brain Theory* 5, 211–55.

MacWhinney, B. (1987) The competition model. In B. MacWhinney (ed.) *Mechanisms of Language Acquisition*. Hillsdale, NJ: Lawrence Erlbaum Associates.

McClelland, J.L. (1989) PDP: Implications for cognition and development. In R. Morris (ed.) *Parallel Distributed Processing: Implications for Psychology and Neurobiology*. Oxford: Clarendon Press.

Nelson, K. (1973) Structure and strategy in learning to talk. *Monographs of the Society for Research in Child Development* 38.

Selfridge, M. (1986) A computer model of child language learning. *Artificial Intelligence* 29, 171–216.

Siskind, J. (1990) Acquiring core meaning of words, represented as Jackendoff-style conceptual structures, from correlated streams of linguistic and non-linguistic input. *Proceedings of the 28th Annual Meeting of the Association For Computational Linguistics*, University of Pittsburgh, Pittsburgh, PA, USA.

2 Representation Issues in Child Language Corpora

KHURSHID AHMAD AND JOHN WRIGHT

This chapter is partly the result of a number of comments made by Edwards (1992) concerning the storage and transcription of child language data, and the subsequent discussion raised by MacWhinney and Snow (1992). The apparent polemic between these authors suggests in our opinion the need for future research into the provision of a formal computational model of child language data, in order to overcome the potential obstacles highlighted by both parties. This paper summarises briefly the principles outlined by Edwards and the comments of MacWhinney and Snow, before proceeding to examine the merit of applying formal computational data modelling techniques to the field of child language data archival. We finish the chapter with examples of the use of relational database modelling in restricted child language domains, in order to highlight the benefits of computational data modelling.

Introduction

In her paper, Edwards (1992) suggests the need for four general principles in archive-based language research:

(i)   Transcribed data must be as readable as possible, and should have a minimum of presentational bias, in order to maximise the possibilities for forming intuitive hypotheses about the data whilst reading through them.

(ii)   Data should be consistently encoded so that a computer search will reveal all occurrences of a particular syntactic, morphological, prosodic or other feature.

(iii)   When analytically categorising features in the data, the categories chosen should contrast systematically, and categories which are not mutually exclusive should be used in conjunction when more than one applies.

(iv)   Data from different sources should be combined only when the methods of elicitation, transcription and encoding are comparable.

MacWhinney and Snow (1992) see Edwards' paper as a direct attack on CHILDES — the CHIld Language Data Exchange System — one of the largest computerised repositories of child language data, and a personal project of theirs. Nearly all of the examples used to justify Edwards' arguments are drawn from data in CHILDES. In essence, MacWhinney and Snow find that much of what Edwards states is erroneous, since it is based on 'confusion' arising from outdated information. This confusion can be summarised as follows:

(i)   Confusion between old (and inconsistent) versions and the current (consistent) version of CHAT (Codes for Human Analysis of Transcripts), the system used for transcribing and encoding child language data in the CHILDES database.

(ii)   Confusion concerning the relationship between the CHAT standard and its actual implementation.

(iii)   Confusion between transcription techniques for automatic analysis and transcription techniques for documentation.

(iv)   Confusion between CHAT guidelines and the larger CHILDES system itself, including the CLAN (Child Language ANalysis) suite of programs.

Edwards' point (ii) and MacWhinney and Snow's corresponding point (ii) are of direct relevance to the discussion below. Edwards can be proved to be correct, in that MacWhinney and Snow's data appears not to be encoded in a yet-to-be-defined standard encoding scheme, but MacWhinney and Snow are perhaps correct to point out that we should distinguish between the CHAT 'standard' and its implementation. Our argument in this paper is that the above points can be more objectively discussed if formal computational data modelling techniques are applied to the domain of child language data. If the underlying data model is grounded on a sound 'semantic' basis, we avoid the need to construct and rely on subjective, biased or overly-specialised child language database systems (by *overly-specialised*, we refer to the number of transcription encoding schemes and data manipulation program suites currently available in the child language domain). The use of conventional database modelling techniques also brings a number of traditional advantages to the field; these will be discussed shortly after a brief discussion of some key concepts in the field of database technology.

It must be stressed that there are two ways of undertaking a critique of a child language corpus: one can either probe the data model itself, or more specifically, the computer representation of that model. This is a confusion pointed out by MacWhinney and Snow in Edwards' paper. Here, we are not attempting to judge the validity of MacWhinney's CHAT data model or indeed any other data model, but are restricting our remarks purely to the field of data representation. We suggest that the application of standard database modelling techniques (such as relational database modelling) will not only eliminate the current disparate collection of separate and incompatible child language data archives, but will also allow future archives to become a standard and, at least computationally, objective means for testing the suitability of the underlying data model.

What is a Database?

A database is defined to be 'a collection of stored operational data used by the application systems of some particular enterprise' (Date, 1986:9). The term *operational data* is used here to distinguish (stored) data in a database from input data, output data or other kinds of data. *Enterprise* is a generic term for any reasonably self-contained human enterprise or organisation, whether scientific, commercial or industrial; it is often referred to as the *application domain*. The term *application systems* refers to the collection of programs for storing and accessing the data. Typically, these programs are designed to be used by several or many users in a given domain, possibly performing different roles.

The organisation of databases appears to be guided by three important working principles, or perhaps, the following three points are emphasised in the literature: firstly, that the operational data of an enterprise may be diverse in nature. For example, in the case of a manufacturing organisation, there may be product data, supplier data, sales data, employee data and so on. Additionally, there is a considerable amount of emphasis on sharing the data among the various components of the enterprise. The second, perhaps consequent, point relates to the notion of data independence — the immunity of applications (user programs) to changes in storage structure and access strategy. This segregation of how data are physically stored or accessed from the applications programs relates to the need of sharing the data among differing users. The third point relates to what is stored in the database in a metaphorical sense. Databases contain a model of the enterprise, or more precisely, a model of the distinguishable indivisible components of the enterprise and how these components interrelate with each other. The 'components' are referred to as *distinguishable objects* or *entities* ('things about which information is to be stored') and include, for example, people, inanimate objects and organisations (of people or objects), and their attributes.

In addition to the entities themselves, the model will also contain information about the *relationships* between the entities. In fact, if we define entities as objects about which information is to be stored in the database, then we may define relationships as a special type of entity. The important point is to stress that relationships are just as important as entities. There is no point designing a model of an organisation with employees and departments if there is no way of linking a particular employee to a particular department.

By constructing a child language database system based on a well-grounded conceptual model, one can address two of the problems indicated by Edwards: firstly, we commit ourselves to a consistent method for transcription and coding of data; secondly, we need not concern ourselves with issues of readability. Child language data may be accessed and displayed or printed in a number of different formats.

Computational Data Modelling

Data modelling can be defined as a set of activities aimed at the derivation of an appropriate database schema for a particular application. A number of different techniques have been employed by computer scientists in order to allow computers to store and represent the knowledge involved in such an application. These techniques can be divided into three general areas: classical data models (such as the hierarchical and network models), neo-classical data models and artificial intelligence (AI) schemata. However, all of these models are based on the same assumptions: computational pragmatism, i.e. that the data structures chosen do indeed reflect the application domain as the analyst sees it; programming expediency, i.e. that the data structures chosen can be supported by the underlying hardware and the available software.

Most modern databases use the relational model (Codd, 1970), one of the so-called neo-classical data modelling techniques. Here, all data and relationships are represented in a database as tables, or *relations*. A relation exists for each entity of interest in the area being modelled. Thus, in child language, there might be relations for studies, children studied, transcript files and so on. In each relation, the rows represent individual occurrences of that entity, while the columns represent specific attributes of that entity. Each row in a relation must be unique; this is achieved by giving the row a unique identifier, known as the *primary key*. Using such identifiers allows the creator of the database to link rows in one relation to rows in another. If a particular row in a relation A is to be related to a row in relation B, this may be achieved by placing the primary key of the row in B as a special attribute in the row of relation A (or vice versa). This special reference attribute is known as a *foreign key*. Relationships between entities in the database are modelled by using foreign keys, or by creating new entities which are used purely to show a relationship — these are termed *relationship relations*.

Relational models, despite their current popularity, are not themselves without fault. The question of relationships between entities has already been mentioned: are relationships to be classified as entities in their own right, or as a peculiar kind of attribute? The relational model also has certain problems representing superordinate and subordinate entities. Recently, and in an attempt to combat this problem, object orientation techniques have been applied to the domain of database technology (Oxborrow, 1989), resulting in the advent of object oriented database management systems (OODBMS). Unlike conventional relational databases where the data are stored separately from the applications programs which access them, OODBMS hinge upon the notion of the *object*, a computational abstraction which incorporates both stored data and process or behaviour. A specific object type, or *class*, consists of a data structure which is used to represent the object, and a number of operations, or *methods*, which can be performed on that object. All communication with the object takes place through these methods, which represent the visible interface of the object class. The object thus controls its own behaviour; no direct access to the internal data structure of the object is allowed. In addition to this, OODBMS provide the facility of object inheritance, where a subordinate object class can be defined which inherits the properties of a superordinate class, but which adds its own special properties. Thus, if an employee object class were defined, then a new object class for managers could be created which inherited the properties of the super-ordinate employee type, and added further fields for data specific to managerial staff.

The AI community has also devoted itself to the study of suitable means of representing knowledge using computer technology, most notably in the form of semantic networks, frames, scripts (Winston, 1992) and connectionist networks (Rumelhart *et al.*, 1986). The latter draws its inspiration from the manner in which it is suggested that knowledge is stored in the neural pathways of the brain; here, computers are used to manipulate matrices of 'units' (representing simplified version of human neurons) which have some local storage capacity and which are highly interconnected. Knowledge is stored in the patterns of weights on these inter-unit connections, and mathematical equations are used to govern the modification of these weights based upon experience of the external world.

The question of how to represent knowledge using a computer is linked to the notion of representation in cognitive science and philosophy, particularly with the work of Fodor and Putnam (Fodor, 1986; Putnam, 1988). Essentially, the choice of which model to use is a philosophical commitment which influences the way the data are used and viewed. Such a choice scopes both the experiments and the observations made. It also introduces artefacts — usually computational objects — into the domain being modelled. This would not be so important if more advanced technology were at our disposal; one can imagine, in the not-too-distant future, a reliable means of data archival where child language is captured at first on digital audio or video tape. This digital data could then be piped through speech recognition and prosodic analysis programs to arrive at a highly formalised machine-readable transcript of the language. Currently, we have only analogue tape and must rely on the speech recognition and prosodic analysis capabilities of human beings, who each have unique (if small) idiosyncrasies in the manner in which they perceive language. The resulting transcripts are therefore highly individualistic and subjective pieces of text, since bias is introduced at many levels during analysis.

A computational model limits this bias. Our suggestion is that by using computational data modelling techniques, we can remove the burden of responsibility for this subjectivity — what Edwards calls 'any assumed relationships of relevance or dependency' — from the shoulders of the developmental psychologist, and formalise it (by placing it in a rigid computational form) so that it may be quantified by all. This would eradicate the need for specific encoding strategies such as CHAT (note that the 'H' stands for 'human'). For all these reasons, it is important that a computational model be chosen which is as objective as possible. An appreciation of this concept is important; it could be suggested that if MacWhinney and Snow had employed a formal computational model from the outset, there would have been no need for the polemic between Edwards and themselves.

Relational Modelling of Child Language Discourse

In order to demonstrate the possible advantages of employing formal database modelling in the domain of child language, we present two examples of relational models. The first represents an attempt to model some of the characteristics of child language data mentioned in Edwards' (1992) paper; the second concentrates on the contextual information surrounding a particular piece of transcribed child language. We begin with a simplified demonstration of how a model may be realised for the underlying data themselves.

There are six documented stages for the development of a relational model. Two of these concern the nature of the data themselves, and ensure that the ranges and types of the data are fully documented. The other four seek to ascertain the entities, attributes and relationships involved in the area under analysis and to combine them into an integrated structure represented by an Entity–Attribute–Relationship diagram. The analyst will begin by documenting the known entities in the application domain.

We may conclude initially that two possible candidates for entity types are *discourse units* and *speech events*. Here, a discourse unit would represent some supra-sentential grouping: a distinct collection of conversational turns which would normally be found as a separate transcript in current archives. Each discourse unit would encompass a number of separate speech units, each representing a clause or group of clauses uttered by an *interlocutor*. The latter would also qualify for status as an entity in its own right. The relationships between these three candidate entities are quite complicated. An interlocutor might at any time be a speaker, an addressee or one of a group of speakers or addressees. Speech events must be related to other (previous or subsequent) speech events, in order to account for what Edwards calls 'time-space iconicity' and 'logical priority'.

The attributes associated with these entities would also necessarily be elaborate. Many of those linked to the speech event entity would correspond to the contextual comments marked by the '%' character in CHAT (MacWhinney, 1991). Typically, we would expect the speech event's attributes to include the speech fragment itself, pointers to the previous and subsequent speech events, the identity of the speaker and addressees, information on such aspects as prosody, gesture and proxemics, a field for extra comments and a unique identifier field (usually a number). The discourse unit entity's attributes would include the following: pointers to the various interlocutors; situational information; links to the speech events associated with the discourse unit; further comments; and a unique identifier field, once again. Finally, the interlocutor entity would contain general information such as names, ages, relationships and so on. Figure 2.1 shows a prototype Entity–Attribute–Relationship diagram for these initial ideas.

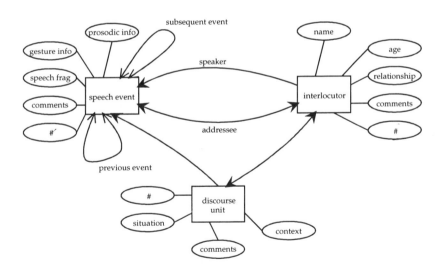

Figure 2.1 An Entity–Attribute–Relationship diagram for a prototype child language discourse model. The attributes labelled with a hash character (#) represent unique identifier fields. Not all of the possible attributes have been placed in the diagram.

We are not attempting to give a complete model for the application domain of child language research, but are presenting some ideas on how child discourse could be modelled using the relational paradigm, in order to show that it could indeed be applicable given further thought.

An example of a relational child language database

In order to illustrate our point further, we have designed and implemented a small prototype child language archive, drawing data from several sources, including studies by Bloom (1973) and portions of corpora such as the Edited Polytechnic of Wales Corpus (Souter, 1989). The database was designed using the relational model, and was created using the Oracle relational DBMS.

Rather than model the underlying structure of the child language data themselves, we concentrated on the contextual information surrounding a particular piece of transcribed child language data. The first stage in modelling any knowledge environment is to ascertain what entities are to be represented in the corresponding model. Here, four specific entities were chosen: *Study, Reference, Subject* and *Output*.

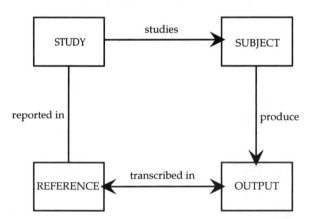

Figure 2.2 An Entity–Relationship diagram for the contextual information surrounding a piece of transcribed child language data. Entities are represented by rectangles, with relationships symbolised by arrows. The presence of an arrow head represents the 'many' side of a relationship; thus there is a many-to-many relationship between Reference and Output, and a one-to-one relationship between Study and Reference.

- *Study.* This entity represents a study carried out at a particular time by one or more psychologists, relating to a particular area of interest and age range.

- *Reference.* This is defined as a database object representing the bibliographical information for a particular study. It contains information on authors, journals, publishers and so on.

- *Subject.* This entity represents an individual child who has been studied for the purposes of gaining insight into the child language acquisition process. It contains general information on the child's background.

- *Output.* This entity contains additional information concerning a piece of transcribed output from a child during a study. This information would include the methodology used, various comments and the filename of the transcript flat file.

Given the above entities, which computationally represent the primitives of transcribed child language utterances, we constructed an Entity–Relationship diagram (Figure 2.2). This diagram, at a certain level of abstraction, gives a visual guide to the entities in a particular data model, and the nature of the relationships between them.

Having defined the entities and relationships in the conceptual model, we specified the attributes associated with each entity in the model. In other words, we decided exactly which information was to be associated with each entity. For example, the *Subject* entity must contain information on the name, sex, race and socio-economic class of the child, as well as information on birth rank (i.e. whether the subject was first-born, second-born and so on), on the relationship of the child with the researcher and on any specific disabilities (blindness, autism, dysphasia, etc.). Figure 2.3 shows the entities and their associated attributes.

Before mapping the conceptual model to tables in a relational database, it was necessary to ensure that a primary key was specified for each entity, so that members of that entity set could be uniquely identified. Rather than choose a subset of the attributes to achieve this, each entity was allocated an additional attribute giving a unique identification number to each of the records in that entity set. Thus, an attribute called Study_number was added to the Study entity, Output_number was added to the Output entity and so on.

The conceptual model was then mapped to tables in an Oracle database. Due to the many-to-many relationship between the Reference and Output entities, it was necessary to create a new entity, called Outref, to represent the relationship: the rules for mapping from a conceptual model to a relational database state that a many-to-many relationship is represented by placing the primary keys of the tables to be linked in a new table — a relationship relation — which contains solely these keys. Having created the tables corresponding to the conceptual model, the database was populated with various examples of child language data as described above.

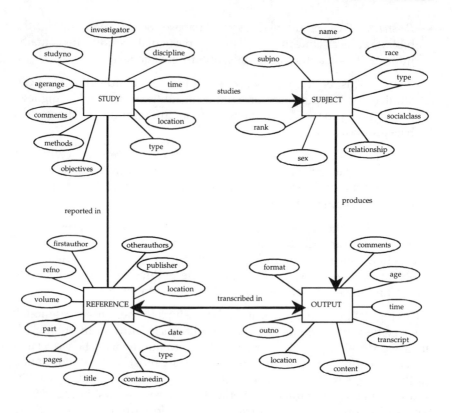

Figure 2.3 An Entity-Attribute-Relationship diagram for the conceptual model of the child language database. Attributes are shown as ellipses.

The resultant database can be queried using SQL (*Structured Query Language*), an ISO standard database language which allows the use to perform queries, obtain reports and create, update and delete tables or even entire databases. The following three queries and output are taken directly from the database and show the power of the relational model and simplicity of the query mechanism:

(1) What references does the database contain for studies of semantic development in children?

```
SQL >  select r.refno, r.firstauthor
       from reference r, study s
       where s.discipline like '% semantic %'
       and s.refno = r.refno
       order by r.refno;
```

Reference Number	First Author
1	Bloom, L.
4	Harris, M.
6	Souter, C.

The SQL query can be 'translated' into English as follows: display, in order of reference number, the reference number and first author of all references in the database which have the same reference number as studies in the database containing the word 'semantic' in the discipline field.

(2) How many blind children have provided transcribed data for the database?

```
SQL >  select count(subject_type)
        from subject
        where subject_type = 'blind';
```

COUNT(SUBJECT_TYPE)

1

This query displays a count of all subjects in the database where the subject_type field is set equal to the word 'blind'.

(3) Which studies carried out in the United States did not take the subject's socio-economic class into consideration?

```
SQL >  select s.investigator
        from study s, subject j
        where s.location like '%USA%'
        and s.studyno = j.studyno
        and j.socialclass is null
        group by s.investigator;
```

Investigator

Lois Bloom

Martin Braine

Melissa Bowerman

Selma Fraiberg

Wick Miller

This query looks for studies containing the word 'USA' in the location field which are linked to subjects whose socio-economic class field has been left blank.

It can be seen that the use of SQL to query such a database has a number of advantages. Most importantly, the language is an international standard, and is known and used by thousands of database users already. The language is also concise and easy to read; the above queries needed little explanation. However, one disadvantage of SQL is that it is usually necessary to have a considerable amount of knowledge regarding the structure of the database, i.e. the underlying relational model in order to formulate queries. This disadvantage can be overcome, however, by developing applications programs which facilitate access to the required data. Most modern DBMS have a large number of facilities for the rapid creation of prototype applications, often based on simple forms and reports templates. Such facilities are normally known as 4GLs (an abbreviation for *fourth generation languages*), and would provide a suitable means to create simple archival and access programs quickly and easily.

Conclusion

With the increasing use of information technology in child language development research, it is becoming more and more important to ensure that a proliferation of separate, highly distinct databases does not arise. The need for a standard, computationally structured method for archiving child language corpora is very much apparent. In this chapter, we assert that such a method is most easily available through the use of computational data modelling techniques, which have already been applied successfully in many scientific and commercial environments. An encouraging sign is the recent proliferation of use of relational modelling in text-oriented domains, such as Tompa and Raymond's (1991) work on database design for dynamic dictionaries, and Kaye's (1988) study of designing databases for the Survey of English Usage. Du Bois and Schuetze-Coburn's (1993) report on the computational representation of syntactic constituent structure as it appears in conversational discourse highlights further the willingness of the linguistic community to turn towards computer technology as a means to represent more precisely the hierarchical nature of language.

It is our opinion that if data modelling of this type is not employed in the future, however, we shall see a rise in the number of separate, incompatible archives with their own suites of customised software. This represents a considerable amount of unnecessary work and can promote inconsistency in an area where the question of transcription and coding of data is already causing problems. This really applies to any research methodology involving information technology. The use of a tried-and-tested method for modelling a complex data environment reduces the initial subjectivity on the part of the data collector, and allows the researcher to use the database as an objective means for testing the utility of a particular theory. Choosing the connectionist paradigm as a basis for research, for example, commits the investigator to a philosophical motivation which is clearly delineated — that the brain is a set of computational processes. Our suggestion here is that by employing the techniques of formal database modelling, we can put behind us the question of the computer representation of the child language data model, and concentrate on using computers as objective probes for the underlying theories of child language development.

References:

Bloom, L. (1973) *One Word at a Time*. The Hague: Mouton.

Codd, E.F. (1970) A relational model of data for large shared data banks. *Communications of the ACM* 13, 377–87.

Date, C.J. (1986) *An Introduction to Database Systems*: Volume 1. Reading, MA: Addison-Wesley. 4th edition.

Du Bois, J.W. and Schuetze-Coburn, S. (1993) Representing hierarchy: Constituent structure for discourse databases. In J.A. Edwards and M.D. Lampert (eds) *Talking Data: Transcription and Coding in Discourse Research*. Hillsdale, NJ: Lawrence Erlbaum Associates.

Edwards, J.A. (1992) Computer methods in child language research: Four principles for the use of archived data. *Journal of Child Language* 19, 435–58.

Fodor, J.A. (1986) *Representations: Philosophical Essays on the Foundations of Cognitive Science*. Cambridge, MA: The MIT Press.

Kaye, G. (1988) The design of the database for the Survey of English Usage. In M. Kytö, O. Ihalainen and M. Rissanen (eds) *Corpus Linguistics, Hard and Soft*. Proceedings of the 8th International Conference on English Language Research on Computerized Corpora. Amsterdam: Rodolpi.

MacWhinney, B. (1991) *The CHILDES Project: Tools for Analyzing Talk*. Hillsdale, NJ: Erlbaum.

MacWhinney, B. and Snow, C. (1992) The wheat and the chaff: Or four confusions regarding CHILDES. *Journal of Child Language* 19, 459–71.

Oxborrow, E. (1989) *Databases and Database Systems: Concepts and Issues*. Bromley: Chartwell-Bratt. 2nd edition.

Putnam, H. (1988) *Representation and Reality*. Cambridge, MA: The MIT Press.

Rumelhart, D.E., McClelland, J.L. and the P.D.P. Research Group (1986) Parallel *Distributed Processing: Explorations in the Microstructure of Cognition — Volume 1: Foundations*. London & Cambridge, MA: The MIT Press.

Souter, C. (1989) *A Short Handbook to the Polytechnic of Wales Corpus*. ICAME, Norwegian Computing Center for the Humanities, Bergen University, P.O. Box 53, N-5027 Bergen, Norway.

Tompa, F.W. and Raymond, D.R. (1991) Database design for a dynamic dictionary. In I. Lancashire (ed.) *Research in Humanities Computing* 1. Oxford: Clarendon Press.

Winston, P.H. (1992) *Artificial Intelligence* (3rd edn). Reading, MA: Addison-Wesley.

3 Arbitrary and Topographic Space in Sign Language Development

JOHN CLIBBENS AND KENNY COVENTRY

The most striking and all-pervasive feature of the natural sign languages used by deaf people is the systematic use of space for grammatical purposes. One example of this is the pronominal system, which relies on the use of pointing to particular locations in space, these locations serving as referential indices in subsequent discourse. Locations may be conventional or arbitrary (in 'syntactic' space), or they may form part of a 'map' of the real world (in 'topographic' space). Verbs in sign language are classified into different classes according to the way in which they use syntactic and topographic space, with 'agreement verbs' inflecting for person and number using arbitrary spatial indices, and 'spatial verbs' inflecting for location in (a representation of) topographic space. There is clearly room for debate as to which of these uses of space are truly syntactic, and which of them should properly be regarded as pragmatic, and this is becoming a focus of discussion amongst sign linguists. Much of the research addressing these issues to date has been conducted on American Sign Language. The present paper reports some preliminary findings of a pilot study aimed at investigating the development of the pronominal reference system in British Sign Language.

Introduction

British Sign Language (BSL), the language of the deaf community in Britain, is one of a large number of natural sign languages that have now been identified around the world (Padden, 1988). These languages share all the structural characteristics of natural spoken languages but differ from the latter in that these structures are realised in the form of visually perceived gestures and other head and body movements, rather than in speech. A consequence of this visual/gestural realisation is that sign languages make systematic use of space to mark grammatical and phonological distinctions.

The phonological system, for example, makes use of sublexical components which are equivalent to the phonological units of spoken language in that they do not carry meaning in themselves, but only when combined to form signs. For manual signs these components take the form of a specific set of handshapes, locations, movements, and hand orientations (in the 'classical' approach to sign phonology originating with the work of Stokoe, 1960; more recent work applying nonlinear models of spoken language phonology to sign language nevertheless retains these basic components at some level). Despite the iconic quality of many signs, which has often been remarked upon (eg the fact that the BSL sign HOUSE involves the hands outlining the shape of a house), there is evidence that signers represent signs mentally in terms of these underlying parameters, rather than as holistic, pictorial, representations. (Here, and below, upper case letters are used to indicate a sign gloss, as is conventional in reporting research on sign language. Hyphens are used where more than one English word is required to gloss a single sign.) Evidence to support the psychological reality of these sublexical parameters comes from the study of errors in sign production (Klima & Bellugi, 1979; see also Clibbens & Harris, 1993, for some remarks on phonological errors and self-corrections in a child acquiring BSL).

The grammar of sign language also makes use of spatial locations and spatial relations. The sign languages that have been studied to date have extremely rich morphological systems involving, for example, the use of distinctive movements to indicate aspectual distinctions in certain verbs (Klima & Bellugi, 1979). The pronominal reference system is a particularly good example of the way in which sign language makes use of spatial location: in both American Sign Language (ASL) and BSL pronouns take the form of pointing gestures. There are conventionalised locations for first and second person reference (with the gesture directed towards the signer and addressee, respectively). Reference to third persons is achieved by associating that person with another point in space. For example, if a signer refers to someone by name, and then points to a location to the right of the signer, that point becomes (temporarily) associated with that person, and subsequent reference can take the form of simply pointing to the same location again. Certain verbs (known as 'agreement' verbs) make use of the same system of spatial locations. These verbs can move between established locations to indicate who is doing what to whom: the verb GIVE, for example, moves between different locations to signify I–GIVE–HER, SHE–GIVES–HIM, and so on.

The use of arbitrarily defined locations in pronouns and agreement verbs, as described above, contrasts with the use of space in another class of verbs (known as 'spatial' verbs). In these verbs movement takes place between locations in a 'map' of real space. The BSL verb MOVE for example can be used to indicate where something is moved from, and where it is moved to, using locations in space which correspond to real locations in the world. In this use of space it would not be possible to arbitrarily employ locations to the left or the right of the signer, the locations employed must stand in the same spatial relation to each other as the real world locations which they represent. The former, arbitrary, use of space has come to be known as 'syntactic' space, the latter, involving the mapping of real locations, as 'topographic' space (Padden, 1990; Bellugi & Klima, 1993).

There is currently some debate within sign linguistics as to the reality of the syntactic/topographic space distinction described above. Liddell, in a series of papers — some as yet unpublished — (Liddell, 1990, 1992, 1994, 1995) has pointed out that, in the first place, agreement verbs (or 'indicating' verbs, as he calls them) and pronouns are not really directed towards a locus, i.e. the actual *point* in space at which reference has been established, but rather to different, specific, heights above it, depending on the individual verb involved. Liddell goes on to distinguish three different types of reference: reference to entities which are physically present at the time of reference, and two distinct kinds of non-present reference — one involving *surrogates* and one involving *tokens*.

Surrogates are entities which are referred to as though they were physically present: in ASL pronouns point at surrogates in the same way that they point towards present referents — normally at chest height. A surrogate is thus to be conceived of as an invisible entity, treated as though it were present and as though it has size, dimensions, and distinguishable body parts. Tokens, according to Liddell, are the product of the process of reference establishment described above, whereby entities are located at specific points in signing space. As already indicated, pronouns and verbs are not directed towards the actual point where reference was established, but to various distances above it. Tokens are not life-size, and cannot be addressed directly (as surrogates can — particularly in reference involving 'rôle-shifting', where the signer takes on the rôle of a participant in the discourse) and they do not seem to have distinguishable body parts, but they are three-dimensional, and not simply points in space. Liddell argues that tokens use space in a less detailed way than surrogates, but that, nevertheless, they do have topographical significance.

Liddell's argument that the so-called syntactic use of space is not entirely non-topographical is well taken. It is clear, however, that there is still a distinction to be drawn here, and one which is supported by both experimental and cognitive neuropsychological evidence (Emmorey,

1992; Poizner, Klima & Bellugi, 1987), even if the terms in which it is drawn need to be rethought.

Liddell (1994) has gone on to suggest that the use of space in ASL is not fundamentally different from the use of space in spoken English. He argues that pronouns and agreement verbs effectively incorporate the use of nonlinguistic gestures within signs, and that this process is similar to the use of pointing and other indicative gestures alongside spoken words. This more recent work of Liddell's involves recourse to a type of mental representation derived from cognitive linguistics — that is, the notion of a 'mental space' (Fauconnier, 1985). This notion has an obvious intuitive appeal if one is seeking an appropriate cognitive representation to mediate between spatial locations in the real world and their representation in a spatially based language; however this very obviousness means that its explanatory potential needs to be carefully evaluated against that of other approaches, such as mental models or propositional representations. One type of mental space which Liddell argues for is a mental representation of the immediate, directly perceivable, physical environment: this type of representation is referred to as 'Real Space'. It is not clear, however, that language users ever operate with such a direct, unselective, representation.

Work on spoken language has clearly demonstrated that knowledge about the functional relationships between objects can override information from immediate sensory experience (Garrod & Sanford, 1989; Coventry, 1992; Coventry, Carmichael & Garrod, 1994). For example, in tasks involving spatial description, it has been demonstrated that contiguity of movement of figure with ground increases the use of the

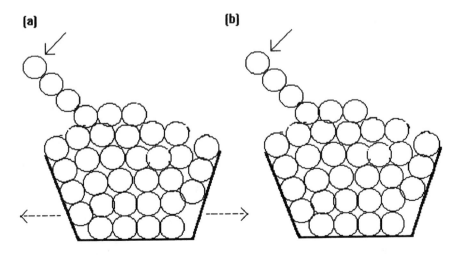

Figure 3.1

spatial preposition 'in': thus Coventry (1992) found that in scenes such as Figure 3.1(a) *in* was used more than in scenes like Figure 3.1(b). Furthermore Coventry *et al.* (1994) found evidence that solids are thought more likely to be contained in bowls than jugs, and, as a consequence, *in* is used more with fruit in a bowl than with fruit in a jug (with high piles of objects). The use of spatial prepositions is thus underdetermined by geometric or topographic information. Such effects may be expected to occur in sign language also. Indicative of this is evidence (Sadalla, Burroughs & Staplin, 1980) that there are asymmetries in judged distance between good reference points and poorer reference points. The distance between a good reference point and a poorer reference point is judged to be less than the distance between the same reference points with the order reversed. With sign language also it is reasonable to predict that the distance between signed representations of figure and ground will be influenced by knowledge about objects and their interactions.

As the examples above make clear, speakers operate with selective representations of what is available to the senses. The choice of a particular 'notation system' for discussing mental representations can often obscure the fact that the form of a representation does not in itself explain how it is that certain entities come to be represented and others do not, or how it is that participants in discourse are able to assume a shared cognitive environment which makes communication possible at all. What seems to be required is a principled account of the way in which different sources of information, including knowledge in long term storage as well as the information currently available to the senses, are drawn on to construct the representations which make communication possible — the precise form of the representation itself may be a far less important matter (cf. Sperber & Wilson, 1986).

The Development of Spatial Reference and Verb Agreement in Sign Language

A number of studies have addressed, in ASL, the acquisition of the system of nominal reference and verb agreement described in the above section (see Bellugi, van Hoek, Lillo-Martin & O'Grady, 1993; Bellugi & Klima, 1993, for reviews). Petitto (1984) looked at the transition from early pointing to the use of similar gestural forms for first and second person reference. She found that the deaf children she studied started pointing at around the same age that hearing children do (9–10 months). This early period was then followed by one in which the children avoided pointing to themselves and other people (while carrying on pointing to objects). When they started pointing to people again, the children made reversal errors, of the type that have been observed in some hearing children: pointing away from themselves to indicate ME, and towards themselves to indicate YOU, before finally mastering the system. Petitto argues that the errors produced by these children, leading to referential forms which are counter-iconic, suggest that the use of pointing as part of the formal reference system of sign language is distinct from other types of referential pointing, providing evidence for discontinuity in the development from prelinguistic gestural communication to language.

Meier (1982) looked at the acquisition of verb agreement, and found that at around two years of age signing children made no use of verb inflections. Thus the utterance YOU(–)GIVE(–)ME would be signed using an uninflected form of GIVE (moving away from the signer) rather than the required agreeing form (moving from the addressee towards the signer). The uninflected form resembles a mime of 'I give you' and would sometimes be accompanied with separate pronoun signs (unnecessary when the inflected form is used). (Note that the use of the uninflected form has the effect of making the sign less iconic.) Between two and three years of age deaf children began to produce forms inflected for verb agreement where the referent was physically present, and where the locations used for the beginnings and ends of verbs would therefore be determined by the actual location of the referent, rather than being arbitrarily assigned. This use was mastered by the age of three, but children made a range of errors during this period, such as providing agreeing forms for verbs which cannot be marked for agreement in adult ASL (e.g. the sign SAY). They would also sometimes inflect a verb like GIVE towards the wrong argument location — leading to an ungrammatical and counter-iconic utterance, but one which indicates that the child is working on a morphological analysis of the sign.

Meier thus demonstrated that children were able correctly to use verb agreement morphology by the age of 3;6, but only where referents were physically present. Prior to this they used uninflected verbs and relied on sign order to make clear the relation between verbs and their arguments — a strategy which produces ungrammatical sentences in terms of adult ASL. Verb agreement for non-present referents, however, does not appear until some time after 4;0, and for most children, not until after 5;0, at around the same time that children become able to establish nominal referents by associating them with spatial loci (van Hoek, Norman & O'Grady-Batch, 1989). Children thus have some knowledge of the use of space early on, but this is restricted to verb agreement for present referents, and they are unable to use spatial loci in other contexts until later.

van Hoek et al. (1989), in a study of nominal establishment and verb agreement in ASL, identify three developmental levels in the referential use of space. They explicitly relate their approach to that of Karmiloff-Smith (1985) on the development of pronominal reference in spoken language discourse. Karmiloff-Smith argues that early on children produce utterances which are correct at the local sentential level, but not integrated at the higher, discourse, level: in a study using a narrative task involving sequences of line drawings the youngest children relied on deictic reference to referents which were physically present, rather than on the anaphoric use of pronouns. Karmiloff-Smith also describes her data in terms of three developmental levels. At Level 1 (mainly four- and five-year-olds) pronouns were only interpretable by reference to the extralinguistic context (the pictures), and there was frequent use of pointing and head and eye movements to support reference. By Level 2 (six- to seven-year-olds) the beginnings of a discourse strategy were emerging: where there was a clear central character (or 'thematic subject') the initial slot was reserved for reference to this character, and pronouns were typically used. Narratives were often less complete at this stage due to the rigid application of this strategy. By Level 3 (eight- to nine-year-olds) there was more flexibility: the initial slot was still preferentially reserved for reference to the thematic subject, but other referents could occupy this slot. Where this occurred it was indicated by the use of differential markers, with the use of pronouns in the initial slot still reserved for the main character.

Karmiloff-Smith explained these results in terms of the spontaneous re-organisation of the child's long-term memory store for referential forms: in line with her 'representational redescription' model of cognitive development (Karmiloff-Smith, 1992). Garrod & Sanford (1988) have argued that the notion of the thematic subject is central to the representation of characters in discourse, with the thematic subject defined as the entity that is focal within the current mental representation of the discourse. (Note that the notion of focus is not in itself sufficient to account for the identification of referents: it is necessary to explain why certain referents are mutually in focus, and how speakers make use of this in constructing interpretable utterances.)

Clibbens (1992) found evidence for a thematic subject strategy in younger children, using a narrative task presented on video. The stories used involved a central character and two more peripheral characters who, nevertheless, played a more extensive rôle in the story than the minor characters in Karmiloff-Smith's stories. With this task children as young as five were found to distinguish between central and peripheral characters, not in the precise way described by Karmiloff-Smith, but in the forms used to refer to characters following an intervening reference to another character. Under these circumstances reference to peripheral characters was normally re-established (using a full NP), but reference to central characters was not. This result is not inconsistent with the general tenor of Karmiloff-Smith's account, but indicates that, if re-organisation is required to allow the choice of different forms for characters of different status, it must have already occurred in the five-year-olds in Clibbens' study.

As noted above, van Hoek et al. (1989) also identify three levels of development in children's use of space for referential purposes in ASL.

They studied 32 children aged 2;4 to 8;11, all of whom were deaf and acquiring ASL as a first language. The task used was a picture story one similar to that of Karmiloff-Smith. The children assigned to Level 1 made no use of space for referential purposes, and did not overtly identify referents. They evidenced no use of referential loci, either for pronouns or verb agreement, and either did not use agreeing verbs, or failed to mark them for agreement. There was no overt identification of central characters. Children at Level 2 used space inconsistently, with inconsistent or unclear identification of referents. Spatialised verb agreement and pronominal reference was haphazard or inconsistent, and identification of referents was also inconsistent. Loci associated with referents would often change arbitrarily (these can change in adult discourse, but such changes are normally motivated). Some agreeing verbs were marked for agreement, but not all. By Level 3 children showed correct and consistent use of space and consistently clear reference.

One point worth noting here is that, while van Hoek *et al*'s three level analysis bears some similarity to that developed by Karmiloff-Smith for spoken discourse, it is less theoretically motivated. Levels 1 and 3 are defined by either no or completely correct use of space, respectively. Level 2 is simply everything in-between. Karmiloff-Smith's Level 2 involved the use of a specific strategy, related to a more general theory, and did not simply represent a transitional state from deictic to anaphoric reference. It is also worth noting that the levels are defined in terms of the simultaneous variation of two distinct factors: the use of space, and the non-spatial identification of referents.

van Hoek *et al.* found that children under three did not use referential loci at all. From three years of age there was an increasing use of referential loci for verb agreement — largely correlated with the non-spatial establishment of reference. By eight years, 75% of narratives showed correct use of spatialised verb agreement, with consistently maintained loci. The correlation between spatialised and non-spatial forms of reference was high — 80% of the narratives could be classified as belonging to one of the three levels — and van Hoek *et al.* concluded that this strong correlation suggests that spatial and non-spatial reference are dependent on the same underlying principles.

The Development of Spatialised Reference in British Sign Language

This section reports on a pilot study which is being carried out to determine whether the same developmental progression can be observed in deaf children acquiring BSL as a first language as that reported by van Hoek *et al.* (1989) for ASL. As far as the authors are aware there has been no previous research on the development of the spatial reference system in BSL. The discussion is limited to the sample of two children (a brother and sister, aged 9 and 7 respectively, from a signing family) that have been studied to date.

The pilot study involves showing the children two videotaped stories recorded using glove puppets. These videos were those used by Clibbens (1992) in a study of the development of narrative reference in hearing children. As indicated above, each video involved a central character and two more minor characters: in one case the central character was a frog and the peripheral characters were teddy bears; in the other the central character was an owl and the peripheral characters were rabbits. In each case the central character plays the rôle of a shopkeeper, and the other characters are customers in the shop. The two parallel versions allow two conditions to be run: a CONCURRENT condition, in which the child watches the story and simultaneously signs it (to the experimenter, who is sitting alongside the monitor on which the video is played back), and a RECALL condition, in which the child first watches the story and then signs it (again to the experimenter, sitting in the same location). In each case the signed stories are recorded for subsequent transcription and analysis. The narrative strategies employed by the two children in the two conditions are summarised below.

GIRL (7) CONCURRENT Condition

— heavy reliance on full nominal forms — reference generally clearly established for this reason

— resorts to null form at times — especially in opening section, when central character alone

— no referential indexing — at one point signs HE (pointing to conventional third person location) but corrects to full form FROG — also two other repairs, both from null form to FROG

— sparse use of directionality in verbs — where it occurs it simply mirrors the direction of the action being watched.

GIRL (7) RECALL Condition

— (story a little confused — some episodes repeated)

— no consistent spatial referential indexing, or spatial agreement with verbs — use of space locally consistent, but switches from one direction to another when repeating same episodes later in narrative

— a lot of null referencing (with no overt referential form) — reference therefore dependent on use of space (which is inconsistent, as noted above)

— several times does not re-establish reference to central character following intervening reference to another character, but always does so with peripheral characters.

BOY (9) CONCURRENT Condition

— more consistent use of space in general — e.g. relative positions of objects (topographic space)

— a lot of null forms — often with rôle-shifting

— consistent use of directional verbs (following direction of action on screen)

— no consistent referential indexing — a lot of re-establishment of reference using full nominal form

— some (limited) use of person classifier predicates.

BOY (9) RECALL Condition

— (episodes a little muddled)

— use of space in directional verbs locally consistent, but inconsistent over entire narrative

— effective use of different locations to distinguish characters locally, but inconsistent overall

— effective use of classifier predicates (using one or two index fingers to represent actors)

— no use of rôle-shifting in this task.

Generally, both children could be said to be at van Hoek *et al.*'s Level 2, but how useful is this classification? Both seem to have a good grasp of the need to identify referents, and are able to do this nonspatially. Both are inconsistent in their use of space across narratives, and neither uses any referential indexing (pointing to an established referential locus) at all. The clear evidence of awareness of the necessity to establish reference in the absence of any spatial indexing suggests that there need not be a close correlation between these two abilities. The classification also fails to pick up differences between the two children: for example, the girl shows indications of a thematic subject strategy, both in her use of reduced forms for the central character, which were subsequently repaired to full nominal forms (in the CONCURRENT condition) and in the fact that she did not always re-establish reference to the central character following an intervening reference to another character (in the RECALL condition), while always doing so for the peripheral characters. In this respect the referential strategies used by the girl resemble those of the five-year-old hearing children in Clibbens' (1992) study. There is no indication of a thematic subject strategy in the boy's narratives (in this respect he resembles the seven-year-old children in Clibbens' (1992) study) but he does make use of rôle-shifting and of predicate classifiers in his narratives, neither of which mechanisms is used by the girl.

Clearly further work is needed in this area of development in BSL. The sample discussed here is very small, and the conclusions drawn above are necessarily tentative. The narrative task used in the present work differs in a number of respects from that employed by van Hoek *et al.* (1989) — in its complexity, and in the use of videotaped presentation rather than line-drawings, for example — and one possible strategy, therefore, would be to use the two tasks together in a larger scale study, in order to pinpoint task-specific effects. Such an approach would parallel work which has demonstrated such task differences with hearing children using spoken English (Karmiloff-Smith, 1985; Clibbens, 1992). Such research also needs to be set in the context of studies directed at spatial representation and spatial reference in adult BSL users.

References

Bellugi, U., van Hoek, K., Lillo-Martin, D. and O'Grady, L. (1993) The acquisition of syntax and space in young deaf signers. In D. Bishop & K. Mogford (eds) *Language Development in Exceptional Circumstances*. Hove: Lawrence Erlbaum Associates.

Bellugi, U. and Klima, E. (1993) Language research: New views of how the brain works. In J. Clibbens & B. Pendleton (eds) *Proceedings of the Child Language Seminar, 1993*. Plymouth: University of Plymouth.

Clibbens, J. (1992) *Comprehension and Production of Discourse Anaphora: A Developmental Study*. Bloomington, IN: Indiana University Linguistics Club Publications.

Clibbens, J. and Harris, M. (1993) Phonological processes and sign language development. In D. Messer & G. Turner (eds) *Critical Influences on Child Language Acquisition and Development*. London: Macmillan; New York: St. Martin's Press.

Coventry, K.R. (1992) Spatial prepositions and functional relations: The case for minimally specified lexical entries. Unpublished PhD thesis, University of Edinburgh.

Coventry, K.R., Carmichael, R. and Garrod, S.C. (1994) Spatial prepositions, object specific function and task requirements. *Journal of Semantics* 11, 289–309.

Emmorey, K. (1992) Processing topographic vs. arbitrary space in ASL. Poster presented at Fourth International Conference on Sign Language Research, San Diego, CA.

Fauconnier, G. (1985) *Mental Spaces: Aspects of Meaning Construction in Natural Language*. Cambridge, MA: MIT Press.

Garrod, S.C. and Sanford, A.J. (1988) Thematic subjecthood and cognitive constraints on discourse structure. *Journal of Pragmatics* 12, 519–34.

— (1989) Discourse models as interfaces between language and the spatial world. *Journal of Semantics* 6, 147–60.

van Hoek, K., Norman, F. and O'Grady-Batch, L. (1989) Development of spatial and non-spatial referential cohesion. Paper presented at Stanford Child Language Research Forum, Stanford, CA.

Karmiloff-Smith, A. (1985) Language and cognitive processes from a developmental perspective. *Language and Cognitive Processes* 1, 60–85.

— (1992) *Beyond Modularity: A Developmental Perspective on Cognitive Science*. Cambridge, MA: MIT Press/Bradford Books.

Klima, E. and Bellugi, U. (1979) *The Signs of Language*. Cambridge, MA: Harvard University Press.

Liddell, S.K. (1990) Four functions of a locus: Reexamining the structure of space in ASL. In C. Lucas (ed.) *Sign Language Research: Theoretical Issues*. Washington, DC: Gallaudet University Press.

— (1992) Tokens and surrogates. Ms., Department of Linguistics and Interpreting, Gallaudet University (to appear in proceedings of the Fifth International Symposium on Sign Language Research, Salamanca, Spain).

— (1994) Conceptual and linguistic issues in spatial mapping: Comparing spoken and signed language. Ms., Department of Linguistics and Interpreting, Gallaudet University.

— (1994) Real, surrogate and token space: Grammatical consequences in ASL. Ms., Department of Linguistics and Interpreting, Gallaudet University. In K. Emmorey and J.S. Reilly (eds) *Language, Gesture and Space*. Hove: Lawrence Erlbaum Associates.

Meier, R. (1982) Icons, analogues and morphemes: The acquisition of verb agreement in American Sign Language. Unpublished PhD dissertation, University of California, San Diego.

Padden, C.A. (1988) Grammatical theory and signed languages. In F.J. Newmeyer (ed.) *Linguistics: The Cambridge Survey, Volume II, Linguistic Theory: Extensions and Implications*. Cambridge: Cambridge University Press.

— (1990) The relation between space and grammar in ASL verb morphology. In C. Lucas (ed.) *Sign Language Research: Theoretical Issues*. Washington, DC: Gallaudet University Press.

Petitto, L. (1984) *From Gesture to Symbol: The Relationship between Form and Meaning in the Acquisition of Personal Pronouns in American Sign Language*. Bloomington, IN: Indiana University Linguistics Club Publications.

Poizner, H., Klima, E. and Bellugi, U. (1987) *What the Hands Reveal about the Brain*. Cambridge, MA: MIT Press.

Sadala, F., Burroughs, W.J. and Staplin, L.J. (1980) Reference points in spatial cognition. *Journal of Experimental Psychology: Human Learning and Memory* 6, 516–28.

Sperber, D. and Wilson, D. (1986) *Relevance: Communication and Cognition*. Oxford: Basil Blackwell.

Stokoe, W.C., Jr. (1960) *Sign Language Structure. Studies in Linguistics, Occasional Papers, 8*. Buffalo: University of Buffalo Press.

4 Do Cross-Sentential Cues to Phrase Structure Facilitate the Acquisition of Syntax?

PENNY FOWLER, JOHN CLIBBENS AND STEPHEN E. NEWSTEAD

Morgan, Meier & Newport (1989) examined the effects of cross-sentential cues to phrase structure following previous findings (Meier & Bower, 1986; Morgan, Meier & Newport, 1987) which suggested that the acquisition of syntax in first language learning is facilitated by language input which incorporates cues to sentence phrase structure.

Using a miniature language methodology, they exposed 3 groups of adult subjects to possible sentences in the language. One group was then exposed to cross-sentential input which incorporated pronominalisation rules into the grammar, the second was exposed to cross-sentential input incorporating permutational rules and the third (control) group was exposed to input containing no cross-sentential cues. Morgan et al. reported that subjects exposed to input incorporating permutational and pronominalisation rules which acted as overt cues to phrase structure were 'completely successful' in learning the syntax whereas those whose input contained no such cue failed to learn complex aspects of syntax.

The present investigation sought to replicate the Morgan et al. (1989) study and produced a reversal of their results. Control subjects acted in the same way as Morgan et al.'s. However, those in the two experimental conditions performed in the opposite direction with the control subjects (who received no cross-sentential cues) performing better on all but one test where no significant differences were found across all three groups. Possible explanations for this finding and criticisms of the relevance and usefulness of a miniature language methodology in shedding light on first language acquisition will be discussed.

Introduction

This study was based directly on Morgan, Meier & Newport's (1989) research which argued that the existence of cues to phrase structure in natural languages is evidence that cues of this nature are *psychologically necessary* for syntax acquisition in that they reduce the load on any possible pre-programming (Chomsky, 1965). Morgan *et al.* stated that 'The predicted extent of pre-programming may be reduced . . . if grammatical structure is clued in input in a fashion that a suitably perceptive learner may exploit' (Morgan, 1986).

In a bid to investigate their claim, Morgan, Meier & Newport (1987), Morgan and Newport (1981) and Meier and Bower (1986), using a miniature language methodology on adult subjects, conducted a series of experiments in which language input incorporated a variety of 'local' cues to constituent structure. The cues used included those of concord morphology, prosody, the use of function words and pronominalisation, all of which can be found in natural languages. They reported that in every case where subjects were exposed to language input which incorporated a cue to phrase or constituent structure, subjects in those groups were able to learn the syntax. Subjects whose input failed to incorporate any such cue were less successful in learning the syntax, particularly the more complex syntax which required knowledge of co-occurrence relations among word classes. They reported that similar results had been found by other researchers (Braine, 1966; Valian & Coulson, 1988).

The present study sought to replicate Morgan *et al.*'s most recent work (1989) using a miniature language methodology in which they introduced 'cross-sentential' cues to phrase structure. Morgan *et al.* proposed that the existence of minimal pairs in close approximation to one another in parental input to young children might supply phrase-structure information cross-sententially. For example, in the parental self-repetition: 'There it is. There's your foot' (Brown, 1973) the proform 'it' may be substituted for the noun phrase 'your foot'. Morgan *et al.* (1989) stated that the proform 'shares the distributional properties of the phrase it has replaced; the fact that a group of words may be replaced by a single word indicates that the group constitutes a phrase'. To discover if cues to phrase structure in the form of proforms would facilitate syntax acquisition, Morgan *et al.* presented subjects with stimulus sets consisting of two sentences accompanied by the same set of geometric referents (a replacement for meaning). The second sentence contained one of two proforms which substituted for one of two different phrases in the first sentence. Morgan *et al.* predicted that the proforms would cue the phrase structure of the paired sentence and that such information regarding phrase structure would facilitate the acquisition of the syntax.

A second experimental condition was included which examined the possible effects of cross-sentential cues to phrase structure in the form of permutations or re-ordering of words where the underlying meaning of the original sentence was retained. Morgan *et al.* noted that 'the fact that a group of words shares a "common fate" across semantically related but differently ordered sentences provides evidence that the group may constitute a phrase'. Subjects were shown two sentences, the second a permuted version of the first. The permuted sentence was generated by a rule allowing for the inversion of two of the phrases within the grammar. Morgan *et al.* predicted that the re-ordering of the second sentence would cue the phrase structure of the first sentence and so provide information which would facilitate the acquisition of the syntax.

Morgan *et al.* reported that cross-sentential cues facilitated the acquisition of syntax. Subjects whose input had not incorporated any cue to phrase structure 'failed to learn the more complex, conditional aspects of syntax' whereas subjects whose input incorporated cues cross-sententially were reported as 'succeeding in learning both unconditional and conditional aspects'.

The following study set out to replicate the Morgan *et al.* (1989) experiment.

Method

Subjects

Forty-two first year undergraduates in Psychology at the University of Plymouth participated as part of a course requirement.

The miniature language

The miniature language used was identical to that described in the Morgan *et al.* 1989 and Morgan & Newport (1981) papers. The Base language upon which the two experimental conditions were founded, could be generated using both phrase structure rules (see Figure 4.1) and using a finite state grammar (see Figure 4.3).

$S \rightarrow AP + BP + (CP)$

$AP \rightarrow A + (D)$

$BP \rightarrow \{ E \}$ or $\{ CP + F \}$

$CP \rightarrow C + (D)$

Figure 4.1 Phrase Structure Rules

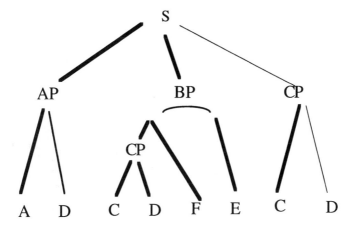

Figure 4.2 Phrase structure tree of sentences of the language. Thicker branches showing obligatory elements; thinner branches denoting optional elements.

(Where S = Sentence, AP = A Phrase, BP = B Phrase, CP = Phrase and where letters A, C, D, E and F = lexical items.)

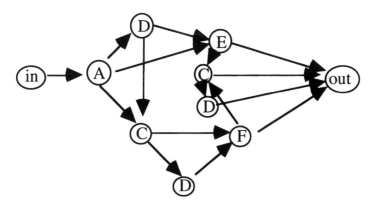

Figure 4.3 State diagram for a finite state grammar of language.

The former gave information regarding the hierarchical nature of the language, in which the language was divided into phrases, A, B and C. This is exemplified in Figure 4.2. The latter enabled sentences to be generated in a linear fashion by moving from state to state as is demonstrated in Figure 4.3. As a result, the language could theoretically be learned either hierarchically or sequentially. Subjects not given any overt cue to phrase structure could still therefore learn the language by learning the possible sequential ordering of words.

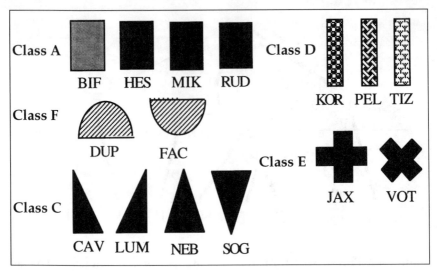

Figure 4.4 Words of the language and their geometric referents.

The three phrases A, B and C were made up of lexical items taken from five form classes analogous to categories like noun, verb etc. The five form classes were labelled A, C, D, E and F and each class contained up to four lexical items (see Figure 4.4).

The language could also be described in terms of a set of conditional and unconditional rules. The unconditional rules described the necessary components of each sentence. For example: 'Every sentence must contain one A word'. The conditional rules captured dependencies between elements within the sentences. Thus the presence of one word might be conditional upon the presence or absence of another. For example: 'If an E word is present, it cannot be preceded by a C word.' (See Table 4.1 for a complete list of the 8 rules of the language.)

Table 4.1 Rules of the language

Rule 1 Every sentence must have at least one *A* word.

| RUD CAV KOR DUP | {A - C - D - F} |
| 'CAV KOR DUP | {C - D - F} |

Rule 2 No sentence may contain more than one *A* word.

| RUD VOT SOG | {A - E - C} |
| 'RUD HES VOT SOG | {A - A - E - C} |

Rule 3 There may be at most one *C* Phrase at the end of a sentence.

| 'BIF VOT LUM TIZ SOG | {A - E - C - D - C} |
| BIF VOT LUM TIZ | {A - E - C - D} |

Table 4.1 *contd*

Rule 4 Every sentence must contain at least one *E or F* word.

      MIK PEL NEB DUP   {A - C - D - F}
      'MIK PEL NEB   {A - D - C}

Rule 5 No sentence may contain more than one *E or F* word.

      MIK SOG DUP NEB   {A - C - F - C}
      'MIK SOG DUP FAC NEB   {A - C - F - F - C}

Rule 6 A *D* word cannot appear after an *E or F* word.

      MIK KOR JAX   {A - D - E}
      'MIK KOR JAX PEL   {A - D - E - D}

Rule 7 A *C* phrase cannot occur before an *E* word.

      'HES NEB JAX SOG   {A - C - E - C}
      HES JAX SOG   {A - E - C}

Rule 8 A *C* phrase must occur before an *F* word.

      'BIF DUP LUM   {A - F - C}
      BIF NEB TIZ DUP LUM   {A - C - D - F - C}

Procedure

Materials and overall presentation

Subjects were divided into three groups: one control and two experimental. Forty of the possible 10,000 base language sentences were used as the input set and presented one by one to each individual subject (see trials below). The input set was selected in exactly the way outlined in Morgan & Newport (1981). Each sentence was projected onto a white screen in front of the subject and appeared for 13 seconds with an inter-stimulus interval of 1.75 seconds. Detail regarding the exact instructions given in the Morgan *et al.* study were not available but a brief description reporting these instructions was followed as closely as possible. Morgan *et al.* stated:

> At the outset subjects were informed that they would see a number of sentences from a miniature artificial linguistic system that included a simple reference world. They were instructed to discover how the words and the figures in this world were paired and to search for patterns in the order and arrangement of words.

The Trials

Trial One

All subjects were shown a single base language sentence per screen.

Above the sentence was a reference field that contained the referents (geometric shapes) of each word.

Trials Two, Three & Four

Subjects were presented with two sentences, one above the other and above both these sentences were the geometric shapes that paired with the top sentence. The top sentence was the same for all conditions and each was taken from the 40 base language sentences.

The sentence shown below the top sentence differed according to condition :

(i)   Base Language Condition

           The second sentence was identical to the first thus acting as a control.

(ii)   Base + Pro-Form

           The second sentence was the same as the first but with the incorporation of a pronoun 'ib' or 'et' to replace either the A phrase or the C phrase. The second sentence was therefore a pronominalised version of the first.

(iii)   Base + Permutation

           The second sentence was the same as the first except that in the second sentence the A and B phrases were placed in reverse order. The second sentence was therefore a permuted version of the first.

The Tests

Tests were given to all subjects, regardless of condition, after each trial. Four different types of test were set:

(i) Vocabulary Tests

These were given after trials 1–3 during which time each of the possible 15 geometric shapes or 'word referents' was projected individually onto the screen directly in front of the subject . Below the shape four lexical items were displayed and were labelled 1–4. Subjects were required to choose which 'word' was paired with the shape shown.

(ii) Rules Tests

These were given after each of the four trials. Each test comprised 32 test items, each item testing one of the eight rules of the language so that each test comprised four test items for each of the eight rules. The test involved showing subjects two sentences, one above the other and labelled 1 and 2 respectively. The two sentences were identical to one another with the exception that one of the two sentences broke one of the eight rules of the grammar and the other did not. In the Morgan *et al.* study 'subjects were requested to indicate which of the two sentences was grammatical'. How this request was actually presented to subjects was not stated. In the present study subjects were asked to decide which of the two sentences 'feel correct according to the patterns in the language you have seen before.'

(iii) Fragment Constituent Tests

These were given after trials 2 and 4. The tests comprised 24 items, each item involving the presentation of two 'fragments', one above the other. The fragments consisted of two or three words taken from permissible sentences in the language. One of the fragments consisted of an intact constituent or phrase (i.e. an A phrase, a B phrase or a C phrase), the other consisted of a fragment from the same sentence but one which cut across two phrases, so violating phrase structure. Subjects were asked to judge which alternative in each pair formed a better 'group or unit'.

(iv) Transformational Constituent Test

Completed after trial 4. The test comprised 24 items, each item involving the presentation of two sentences, one above the other. The sentences were taken from permissible sentences in the base language but both sentences were permuted. One was permuted in such a way that phrase structure was preserved, the other so that phrase structure was violated. No item shown was the same as any sentence shown to subjects in the Permutation Condition. Subjects had to judge which set was preferable.

Results

Vocabulary Tests

In the Morgan *et al.* study, all subjects with the exception of four (whose data were discarded) had reached ceiling on the last vocabulary test. In the present study only 11 out of 14 subjects scored perfectly in the Base Language condition, only seven scored perfectly in the Proform condition and only five scored perfectly in the Permuted condition. Allowing for a single error, all subjects in the control condition passed at this standard whereas only eight subjects in the Proform and nine in the Permuted condition achieved this standard. These results made further comparisons between the two studies problematic if the same criterion for inclusion were to be applied as that used by Morgan *et al.* In response to this problem, analysis of the remaining tests' data was carried out, firstly using all subjects and secondly using data from subjects who scored at least 14 out of 15 on the Vocabulary Tests.

Rules Tests

Morgan *et al.* presented results from trials 2–4 and trial 4 on its own. Table 4.2 shows their mean scores for these trials compared to the mean scores of subjects in the present study using all subjects data.

Table 4.2 A comparison of results on Rules Tests trials 2–4 and trial 4

	Total Rules Test Scores			
Condition	*Mean (Fow)*	*Mean (Mor)*	*SD (Fow)*	*SD (Mor)*
Base				
Trials 2–4	64.2 (64.2)	63.56	9.35	8.34
Trial 4	21.2 (21.2)	21.56	3.88	3.21
Proform				
Trials 2–4	52.5 (53.1)	77.44	5.25	12.44
Trial 4	17.5 (17.37)	26.89	2.84	4.68
Permuted				
Trials 2–4	56.85 (58.4)	76.00	7.23	7.28
Trial 4	19.4 (20.1)	27.78	3.99	3.35

('Fow' = results from the Fowler *et al.* study; 'Mor' = results from Morgan *et al.* (1989) study. SD = standard deviation.) (Data from subjects who scored to criterion in the Vocabulary Tests are shown in brackets.)

Results of this chapter show an opposite trend to that appearing in the Morgan *et al.* study although the Base language condition scores remain virtually identical for both trials 2–4 and trial 4. When all subjects' data was analysed, a main effect of condition was found $F(2,39) = 8.91$, $p < 0.001$. Follow up analysis showed that subjects in the Base language condition performed significantly better than those in the Proform condition ($p < 0.001$) and significantly better than those in the Permuted group ($p < 0.05$) on trials 2–4. On trial 4 alone the Base was better than the Proform ($p < 0.05$). When separating results according to unconditional and conditional rules on trials 2–4 and trial 4 using all subject data a main effect of condition was found on the unconditional rules, $F(2,39) = 8.42$, $p < 0.001$ on trials 2–4. Follow up analysis showed the Base language condition performed better than the proform and permuted groups, both at $p < 0.01$.

On trial 4, a main effect of condition was again found $F(2,39) = 4.3$, $p < 0.05$. Follow up analysis showed that the Base group performed better than the Proform at $p < 0.05$. When data was discarded, the Base language group scored higher than the two experimental groups although the difference was no longer significant. For the conditional rules, no differences were found in the performances by subjects from the three conditions.

Fragment Constituent Tests

The results for both studies were similar in that no differences between groups were found on either of the two tests with the exception of the Morgan *et al.* study where the Permuted group scored significantly better than the Base Language group on the second test only, $F(1,24) = 5.20$, $p < 0.05$. Only the Permuted group scored above chance in the Morgan *et al.* study. The Proform group scored above chance on the first trial only in the Fowler *et al.* study.

Transformational Constituent Test

The two studies' results were similar in that no significant differences were found between groups. Only the experimental groups scored significantly above chance on this test in the Morgan *et al.* study.

Discussion

The most remarkable finding of the present study was the almost complete reversal in trends on the rules tests (tests of syntax acquisition) when compared with the results of the Morgan *et al.* study. The present study found that subjects in the Base language condition performed virtually identically to the equivalent subjects in the Morgan *et al.* study, yet the Proform and Permuted condition groups whose input incorporated cues to phrase structure performed at best no better than the Base condition, and at worst significantly worse than the Base condition: the opposite effect to that reported by Morgan *et al.* Tests of phrase structure revealed that subjects whose input incorporated cues to phrase structure acquired no more information pertaining to that structure than subjects lacking this extra information. This point is central to the claims made by Morgan *et al.* If knowledge of phrase structure is necessary for syntax acquisition and the Proform and Permuted groups had not fully acquired the phrase structure then the results on the rules tests in the present study are to be expected. Indeed, subjects in the Proform and Permuted conditions may have been hindered rather than helped by their input. These subjects had three tasks to attend to: matching of word to referent shape, looking for patterns in the sentences and observing the second sentence and how it related to the first. Subjects in the Base condition had only two tasks: the first two outlined above.

The evidence so far would seem to support the findings of the Fowler *et al.* study. However, it is possible that other factors might account for the difference in findings. The procedure outlined in the original study was followed as closely as possible with the exception of one difference in the Rules Test instructions. The Morgan *et al.* study stated that 'subjects were requested to indicate which of the two sentences is grammatical'. In the present study subjects were asked to 'Judge which of these sentences you feel is correct according to the patterns in the language you have seen before.'

A study on artificial language learning (Reber *et al.*, 1980) reported that the type of instruction given can affect performance. In particular a difference in ability to make grammaticality judgements was reported when instructions were either implicit or explicit. Either type of instruction can facilitate performance but under differing conditions. The addition of the word 'feel' into the instructions may have inadvertently encouraged subjects to base their judgements on their implicit or intuitive judgments about the task rather than encouraging them to make conscious, explicit, rule judgements as might have been made in the original study. In the light of this possibility, a second study is currently in progress examining effects of differing instructional conditions on rule learning.

The question of the usefulness of a miniature language methodology in throwing light on first language acquisition processes has been frequently defended (Morgan & Newport, 1981; Morgan *et al.*, 1987; Meier & Bower, 1986; Brooks *et al.*, 1993). The present study's findings might serve to question the appropriateness of this methodology. The fact that two virtually identical procedures produced such different results might serve to indicate that even subtle changes can strongly affect outcome. Such procedural changes, for example in the type of instruction given, might be more relevant to the circumstances under which adult second language acquisition takes place. Also, the effects of different learner strategies, so commonly documented in second language learning research, further indicate that this methodology might be more appropriate to the study of second language acquisition.

It seems unlikely that one simple instruction can have made such a difference to the results but this finding does cast doubt on the usefulness of this technique in throwing light on natural acquisition processes. Perhaps, as stated above, this finding sheds light on the factors which might influence adult second language acquisition and with this possibility in mind, we aim to continue this investigation.

References

Braine, M.D.S. (1966) Learning the positions of words relative to a marker element. *Journal of Experimental Psychology* 72, 532–40.

Brooks, P.J., Braine, M.D.S., Catalano, L., Brody, R.E. and Sudhalter,V. (1993) Acquisition of gender-like noun subclasses in an artificial language: The contribution of phonological markers to learning. *Journal of Memory and Language* 32, 76–95.

Brown, R. (1973) *A First Language*. Cambridge, MA: Harvard University Press.

Chomsky, N. (1965) *Aspects of the Theory of Syntax*. Cambridge, MA: MIT Press.

Meier, R.P. and Bower, G. H. (1986) Semantic reference and phrasal groupings in the acquisition of a miniature phrase structure language. *Journal of Memory and Language* 25, 492–505.

Morgan, J.L. (1986) *From Simple Input to Complex Grammar*. Cambridge, MA: MIT Press.

Morgan, J.L., Meier, R.P. and Newport, E.L. (1987) Structural packaging in the input to language learning: Contributions of prosodic and morphological marking of phrases to the acquisition of language. *Cognitive Psychology* 19, 498–550.

Morgan, J.L., Meier, R.P. and Newport, E.L. (1989) Facilitating the acquisition of syntax with cross-sentential cues to phrase structure. *Journal of Memory and Language* 28, 360–74.

Morgan, J.L. and Newport, E.L. (1981) The role of constituent structure in the induction of an artificial language. *Journal of Verbal Learning and Verbal Behavior* 20, 67–85.

Reber, A.S., Kassin, S. M., Lewis, S. and Cantor, G. W. (1980) On the relationship between implicit and explicit modes in the learning of a complex rules structure. *Journal of Experimental Psychology: Human Learning and Memory* 6, 492–502.

Valian, V. and Coulson, S. (1988) Anchor points in language learning: The role of marker frequency. *Journal of Memory and Language* 27, 71–86.

5 Preverbal Communication in Young Children with Down's Syndrome: The Use of Pointing and Other Gestures

FABIA FRANCO AND JENNIFER WISHART

Introduction

In this study some aspects of communication in young children with Down syndrome (DS) were investigated. It is known that virtually all of the major developmental milestones are delayed in appearance by DS. Language acquisition poses specific problems, however, with children typically scoring significantly lower on language tests than would be expected on the basis of overall mental age. This notwithstanding, DS children are typically portrayed as interested in interacting with other people and as very sociable. In the continuing absence of language, non-verbal communication must therefore remain an important means of communication for much longer to them than for non-delayed (ND) children.

In normal development it is known that language acquisition is firmly rooted in earlier, non-verbal communicative behaviours. One aspect of prelinguistic communication that has recently received a lot of attention is the gestural one, particularly the gesture of pointing.

Pointing is considered by many theorists to be specifically relevant to language development. In a series of experimental studies, Franco & Butterworth (in press) have shown that in ND 10–24 month olds the 'core meaning' of pointing is a referential-declarative one: it is a gesture used to share attention and internal states about a specific object with another. In a certain sense, this promotes the conditions for the development of the conventional and propositional aspects of linguistic communication, used to accomplish the declarative function.

Pointing emerges around one year of age together with the imperative-instrumental gesture of reaching. Reaching and pointing gestures can be clearly distinguished from each other by the production contexts and by some important co-occurring non-verbal behaviours, such as the pattern of visual checking of the partner associated with each. Later, pointing can also be used with an imperative, requesting function, e.g. to induce another to give a desired, out-of-reach object.

Interestingly, it has been shown (Baron-Cohen, 1989) that autistic children effectively do not produce nor comprehend declarative pointing, although they seem to have no problems with imperative gestures. There are no systematic studies of DS children on this issue. It has however been found that DS children do have specific difficulties in producing pointing gestures with an imperative-instrumental function (Mundy *et al.*, 1988) — a difficulty *opposite* to that of autistic children. In the present study we therefore investigated non-verbal communication in DS children, with special attention to the pointing gesture. It seemed probable that pointing might follow different developmental pathways in DS and ND children.

The second point we addressed in this study was the effect of different types of social partner on communication, specifically the mother and an agemate. In general, the literature on this subject shows a more advanced pattern of communication when babies and young children are interacting with an adult, mainly because of the 'scaffolding' provided by the adult but not by an agemate. However, children do spend time with and experience interacting with agemates. Therefore, we aimed to clarify the features of child–child interactions and any specific contribution these might make to the development of communication.

The role of the communicative partner is also relevant to theories of the origin and function of the pointing gesture in communication. In one of the prominent theories about the origin of pointing, Vygotsky's (1962), pointing serves to replace failed reaching to a desired out-of-reach object. In such situations, the 'competent' (i.e. able to help the baby to gain the object) adult would point to the object and the baby would learn to use the gesture instrumentally herself — a function later carried out by language. Another theory, originally put forward by Millicent-Shinn (1900), claims that pointing initially has an informative function. Bruner (1983), for instance, suggests that pointing is a non-verbal sign for a 'what's that?' question, to which the adult responds by providing the name of the object pointed to.

If either of these theories is correct, in the early stages of pointing development the production level should drop when the partner is an agemate, that is, someone who is in no better position than the baby to gain an unreachable object or to make it work for the baby, nor able to provide verbal labels or enriching communications. However, if instead pointing has a referential-declarative function, one of sharing internal states concerning the external reality with another, the gesture should also be observed in agemate communication.

Given that pointing has been shown to be specifically related to language development, interacting with an agemate may give an important contribution to the consolidation and development of communication. This is a relevant point when we think how we might enrich the environment/experience for children who have particular difficulties in language development, such as children with DS.

Method

Children and mothers attended the laboratory in twos. Sessions were videorecorded.

Subjects

22 children (14 girls and 8 boys) with DS aged 21–47 months (M = 37.25; SD = 6.8). Karyotype information was available in all cases; all children were standard Trisomy 21, with one also showing a small percentage of XXX cells. The sample comprised 75% of all children with DS within the targeted age band who resided within the Lothian region of Scotland, and was representative of the wider DS population in respect to all relevant population variables.

All subjects had been volunteered by their parents in response to a request initially made by either the local Down's Syndrome Association (DSA) or by a professional involved with the family. The majority of children were strangers to each other. All but 2 subjects attended either a playgroup or nursery on a regular basis.

Procedure

Experimental session: subjects were tested first in the mother–child and then in the child–child conditions. In both conditions, children were presented with two communicative contexts, each lasting for 3 minutes:

(*dolls*) 'declarative-referential' context, in which two remotely controlled, animated dolls, 2.5 metres away, moved or were stationary, in alternating 7 second cycles;

(*toys*) 'imperative-instrumental' context, in which toys were demonstrated by the experimenter and then placed just out-of-reach on the table top.

Communication level: This was assessed using the Expressive Scale of the *Reynell Developmental Language Scales* (Rey/exp) — a direct test of the child's expressive language capabilities and the Communication Scale of the *Vineland Adaptive Behavior Scales* (Vin/exp) — a maternal report scale which gives an overall measure of language level plus a breakdown into expressive and receptive components.

Cognitive level: 6 standard trials of a Stage V–VI (invisible displacement) object concept task were presented, followed by a set of trials in which chocolate rather than toys were hidden.

Data analysis

Children with DS were divided into three groups on the basis of (a) chronological age, (b) Vin/exp age level, and (c) Rey/exp age level, in order to allow developmental analyses (see Table 5.1). The reported age divisions were chosen to allow direct comparisons with data of ND infants reported by Franco & Butterworth (in press).

Table 5.1 Grouping of children with DS on the basis of chronological age, Vineland/expressive age level, and Reynell/expressive age level. Age level expressed in months

	Chronological age	Vineland/expressive	Reynell/expressive
(I)	31–36 months (N = 10)	12–15 months (N = 7)	< 12 months (N = 9)
(II)	37–42 months (N = 7)	16–19 months (N = 4)	12–15 months (N = 6)
(III)	43–48 months (N = 5)	20–24 months (N = 9)	16–19 months (N = 5)

Reported analyses concern:

(1) mean frequency of gestures: pointing (arm and index finger extended), indicating (arm extended and non-conventional indicating hand postures), reaching (arm extended and palm downward in a grasp posture), and 'others' (e.g. clapping, ciao, all-gone etc.). As children with DS were found to make frequent use of a 'give me' gesture (palm extended upwards, fingers opening and closing) — a gesture infrequently used by the ND subjects in the same experimental contexts, and not a standard Makaton sign (a signing system based on British Sign Language) — these gestures were added into the reaching category for all analyses since they clearly served the same function as reaching, i.e. requesting.

(2) mean proportion of gestures associated with visual checking of the partner. The 'locus' of checking with respect to the gesture was also analysed: gestures were classified according to the timing of first look to the partner within a time window extending from 2 seconds before gesture initiation ('before'), during gesture execution ('during'), and 2 seconds after gesture completion ('after'). A gesture was classified as associated with multiple checking when a look to the social partner occurred on at least two occasions (e.g. before and during gesture).

Interobserver reliability was 0.79 (Cohen's *k* corrected for chance).

Results

The assessment of communicative skills and cognitive status could not be carried out with the first 2 subjects. Therefore, the following results are based on a sample N = 20:

Reynell: 9 children failed to pass any Rey/exp item, scoring < 12 months. Mean score for the remaining 11 children was 16.5 months (SD = 3.7).

Vineland: mean score was 18.5 months (SD = 4.5). More specifically, mean receptive score was 23.0 months (SD = 10.1) and mean expressive score was 17.6 months (SD = 4.0).

Object concept task: Only 2/20 subjects succeeded on all 6 Stage V–VI trials.

Data are presented for mother–child condition, followed by child–child condition. DS data are then compared with equivalent data sets from Franco & Butterworth studies with ND infants, using Rey/exp and Vin/exp age levels to match for developmental level. Because of difficulties experienced in the imperative-instrumental context (out-of-reach toys) in the child–child condition (e.g. the two agemates often became more involved in playing with each other than in attending the out-of-reach toys being presented), complete data were available for the mother–child condition only.

Mother–child condition

Gestures. Analyses of variance carried out on mean frequency of pointing, indicating, reaching (also including 'give-me') and other gestures (e.g. clapping, ciao, all-gone etc.) produced in the two contexts (dolls/toys) showed a significant gesture x context interaction ($F[2,32]=28.5$, $p < 0.0001$): see Figure 5.1.

Pointing was more frequent in the context of dolls than toys, with reaching restricted mainly to the toy context; indicating and other gestures were more common in the doll context. This indicates that children with DS show differentiated intentions in the doll (declarative-referential) *vs* toy (imperative–instrumental) contexts: declarative communication was served mainly by pointing whereas imperative communication was served mainly by the reaching gesture.

Visual checking. Data consisted of the proportion of gestures associated with a look to the partner either 'before', 'during', or 'after' the gesture. Analysis of variance of visual checking showed an increase of checking with age ($F[2,16]=3.7$, $p < 0.05$) and a significant interaction between gesture and locus ($F[4,64]=2.7$, $p < 0.04$): see Figure 5.2.

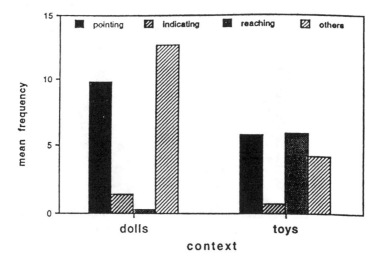

Figure 5.1 DS Mother–Child: Gesture x context (F2, 32 = 28.5, p < 0.0001).

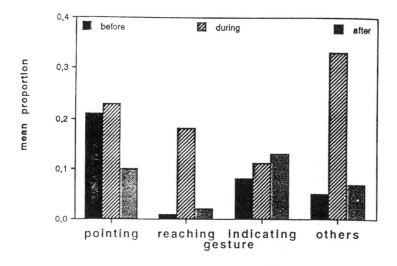

Figure 5.2 DS Mother–Child: Gesture x locus of checking (F4, 64 = 2.7, p < 0.04).

Different gestures had different patterns of associated visual checking. Whereas all gestures show high proportions of checks 'during' gesture execution, only in the case of pointing was a similarly high proportion associated with 'before' checks.

Checking 'during' gestures is typically interpreted as an indicator of

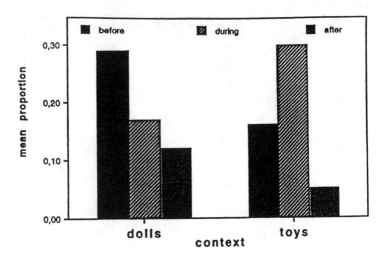

Figure 5.3 DS Mother–Child Pointing: Locus of checking x context (p < 0.06).

intentional comunication. The above patterns of checking are identical to those found in ND infants (see below) and can be interpreted as evidence that only in the case of pointing (with its associated 'before' checking) do children show awareness that the attention of the partner is a necessary precondition for the goal of pointing (a declarative one: to share 'something' about a common referent) to be achieved: here, the partner's 'mind' itself is part of the goal. In contrast, reaching does not need checking 'before' to achieve its goal (an imperative one): here, the partner is only a means to achieve the real goal, i.e. the object (Camaioni, 1992).

Finally, only pointing showed a significant shift in the locus of checking according to context: see Figure 5.3.

In the declarative–referential (dolls) context, pointing was characteristically associated with checking 'before' the gesture whereas in the imperative–instrumental (toy) context, 'during' became the more common locus of checking, as in reaching. This suggests that pointing may also serve an imperative function in the toy context.

Comparison with child-child condition

We recall that comparisons are possible only for the declarative–referential (dolls) context (see p. 56). Only results differentiating mother–child (MC) and child–child (CC) conditions are reported here.

Gestures. Analysis of variance carried out on gesture occurrence showed that there was a higher frequency of gestures in the mother–child than in the child–child condition (F[1,16]=5.8, p < 0.03): see Figure 5.4.

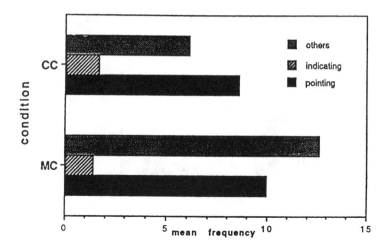

Figure 5.4 DS Mother–Child *vs* Child–Child: Gesture x partner (F2, 32 = 6.1, p < 0.006), Partner (F1, 16 = 5.8, p < 0.03).

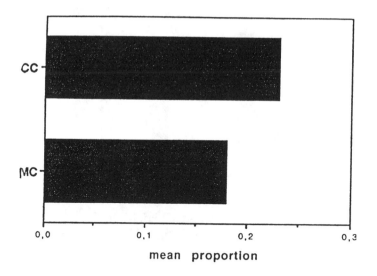

Figure 5.5 DS Mother–Child *vs* Child–Child: Partner x checking p < 0.06).

A significant gesture x condition interaction (F[2,32]=6.1, p <0.006) revealed that twice as many other gestures were produced in the mother-child as in child-child context.

Visual checking. Again, the pattern of checking associated with gestures

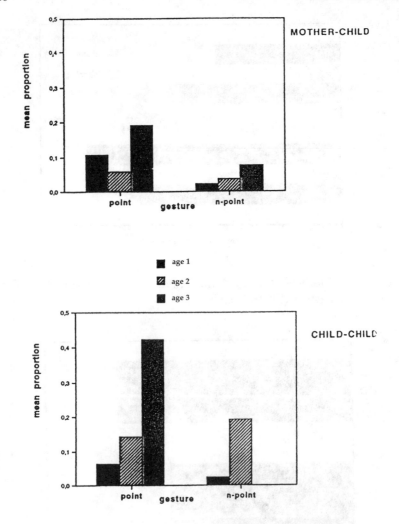

Figure 5.6 DS Mother–Child *vs* Child–Child: Multiple checking x gesture x age (M–C: gesture F1, 16 = 4.5, p < 0.05), C–C: gesture x age F2, 19 = 8.5, p < 0.002).

was similar in the two conditions, but there was a tendency for a higher proportion of gestures to be associated with checking in the child–child (0.23) than in the mother–child condition (0.18): see Figure 5.5.

This trend did not reach full significance (p <0.06) but suggests that children may have felt a greater need to check with an agemate, either because of lack of familiarity, or because of the more limited linguistic feedback provided by the agemate.

This hypothesis is further supported by the analysis of multiple checking. Whereas the mother–child analysis simply revealed that pointing is associated with multiple checking significantly more than non-pointing gestures independently from age, the child–child analysis showed that multiple checking with pointing at age 3 was three times more frequent than at younger ages and was no longer found in association with other gestures (F[2,19] = 8.5, p< 0.002). Figure 5.6 highlights how children's responses differed according to which type of partner was involved in the interaction, with multiple checking more commonly used when pointing for an agemate than for the mother.

Comparisons with normative data

Comparisons are based on Reynell and Vineland expressive levels of children with DS and are limited to ND data sets available from Franco & Butterworth (in press; Franco, Perucchini & Butterworth, 1992). Only results highlighting DS/ND differences are reported here.

Mother–child condition

Ss groupings were as follows: 12–15, 16–19 months for bothVin/exp (N = 11) and Rey/exp levels (N = 11) for subjects with DS, and CA for ND subjects (N = 25).

Gesture. No population related difference was found in the way in which pointing and reaching were characteristically distributed in the declarative–referential (dolls) and imperative–instrumental (toys) contexts. However, a population x age level x context x gesture analysis of

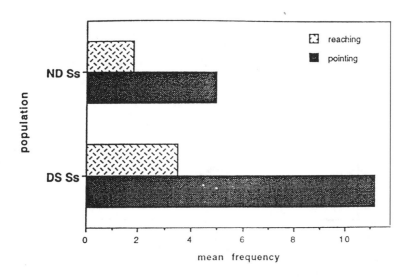

Figure 5.7 Mother–Child DS Ss *vs* ND Ss: Population x gesture (F1, 32 = 10.9, p < 0.002).

variance showed that children with DS produced twice as many gestures as ND subjects (F[1,32] = 10.9, p < 0.002): see Figure 5.7.

This was due to children with DS pointing significantly more often than ND Ss (p < 0.004). These results suggest that despite the age differential between the two samples, pointing and reaching were used for similar communicative purposes in the two groups but with DS Ss making much more frequent use of gestures in communicating.

Visual checking. No population-related differences were found in the relationship between gesture and the timing of any associated visual checking of the partner.

Child–child condition

Subjects groupings were as follows: 12-15, 16-19, 20-24 months (Vin/exp, N = 20); 12–15, 16–19 months (Rey/exp, N = 11) for children with DS; CA for ND infants (N=32).

Gesture. In the analysis of variance based on DS Vin/exp levels, children with DS produced over twice as many gestures (5.8) as ND infants (2.3) (F[1,46] = 8.55, p < 0.005), as in the mother–child condition. Results were similar in the analysis based on DS Rey/exp levels.

Visual checking. In the analysis of variance based on DS Vin/exp levels, there was a tendency for a higher proportion of pointing gestures to be associated with checking in DS than in ND subjects (0.23 vs.16). Moreover, there was an effect of population on the developmental pattern of checking with pointing (F[4,92]=2.4, p < 0.05): see Figure 5.8.

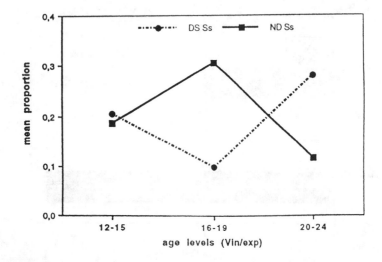

Figure 5.8 Child–Child DS Ss *vs* ND Ss: Checking 'before' pointing: Population x age (F4, 92 = 2.4, p < 0.05).

Whereas checking 'before' pointing peaked at 16–19 months for ND infants, it did so at 20–24 months for children with DS. More specifically, only children with DS showed a preference for checking 'before' rather than 'during' or 'after' pointing at 20–24 months (p < 0.003). This may derive from a replacement of checking 'before' by language in ND infants but not in children with DS: for them, checking 'before' pointing remains the main way to ensure that the partner is attending. Similar results were obtained in the analysis based on DS Rey/exp levels.

Conclusion

The main population difference indicated a more extended use of gestures in young children with DS than ND infants. However, children with DS used pointing similarly to ND subjects: primarily as a declarative–referential gesture aimed at sharing with a social partner some internal state (e.g. surprise) aroused by (and about) an event. In imperative–instrumental communicative contexts, the imperative aim of getting the social partner to provide the desired toy is achieved by reaching and, specific to children with DS in our studies, by 'give-me' ritualised gestures. Considering the more extended use of gestures in children with DS, the fact that we obtained a pattern similar to ND subjects in the imperative-instrumental context only by combining reaching and 'give-me' gestures may be an indication of some difficulty in requesting in children with DS. Moreover, it seems to suggest a developmental difficulty opposite to that of autistic children, whose problem lies in declarative–referential communication (Baron-Cohen, 1989; Mundy et al., 1988; Sigman et al., 1986).

It is also important that no main differences emerged in child-child interaction between DS and ND subjects: even though they may produce fewer gestures than when with their mothers, with an agemate (i.e. a person with their linguistic/cognitive competence), children with DS, if anything, seemed *more* aware of the requirements for successful communication, as evidenced by their advanced checking patterns. We suggest that the agemate is a 'difficult' but stimulating partner for ND babies and young children with DS: the lack of 'scaffolding' and the poverty of feedback with respect to an adult make the baby/child more aware of the other. It somehow obliges the young child to make recourse to her/his higher level resources. An implication of such interpretation is that the agemate lies in the 'proximal development zone' for some aspects of the developing communication system.

On the whole, these results suggest that the longer time spent by children with DS interacting with people before language emerges gives them the opportunity to 'specialise' in preverbal communication. They are not just delayed in language acquisition because of their cognitive handicap: they follow a different path, that of specialised preverbal communication.

Acknowledgements

Support by ESRC (UK) R000231286 grant to F. Franco and by MRC (UK) G9011079N Project Grant to J. Wishart; travel and exchange funds from MPI 40% (I), C.N.R. (I) 92.04355.CT08 grant, and from the University of Edinburgh. Comparison data from the above mentioned ESRC grant to F. Franco and G. Butterworth. Further details about this study are published in Franco & Wishart (1995).

References

Baron-Cohen, S. (1989) Perceptual role-taking and protodeclarative pointing in autism. *British Journal of Developmental Psychology* 7, 113–27.

Bruner, J.S. (1983) *Child's Talk: Learning to Use the Language.* Oxford: Oxford University Press.

Camaioni, L. (1992) Mind knowledge in infancy: The emergence of intentional communication. *Early Development and Parenting* 1, 15–22.

Franco, F. and Butterworth, G. (in press) Pointing and social awareness: Declaring and requesting in the second year. *Journal of Child Language.*

Franco, F., Perucchini, P. and Butterworth, G. (1992) Pointing for an agemate in 1-2 year olds. Paper presented at the *Vth European Conference on Developmental Psychology,* Sevilla, September.

Franco, F. and Wishart, J. (1995) Use of pointing and other gestures by young children with Down syndrome. *American Journal of Mental Retardation* 100 (2), 160–82.

Mundy, P., Sigman, M., Kasari, C. and Yirmiya, N. (1988) Nonverbal communication skills in Down syndrome children. *Child Development* 59, 235–49.

Millicent-Shinn (1900), quoted in R.H. Schaffer (1984) *The Child's Entry into a Social World.* London: Academic Press.

Sigman, M., Mundy, P., Sherman, T. and Ungerer, J. (1986) Social interactions of autistic, mentally retarded and normal children and their caregivers. *Journal of Child Psychology and Psychiatry* 27, 647–56.

Vygotsky, L. (1962) *Thought and Language.* Cambridge: Cambridge University Press (first published in 1926).

6 Negative Feedback in Language Addressed to Hearing-impaired Children

CLARE GALLAWAY AND MARGARET JOHNSTON

Negative Feedback in Speech Addressed to Hearing and Hearing Impaired Children

Children's early language frequently includes utterances like this:

I maked it with water (Sarah, 4;5. Brown, 1973)

How do children manage to retract from such errors? If, as Brown & Hanlon (1970) suggest, parents correct children's factual errors but not their grammatical ones, children appear to learn the rules of their language without the support of negative evidence to guide their hypotheses about grammar. Evidence from more recent studies would suggest that a wider evaluation of parental response patterns may yet reveal differential responses to well-formed utterances (WFUs) and ill-formed ones (IFUs) (Hirsh-Pasek, Treiman & Schneiderman, 1984; Demetras, Post & Snow, 1986; Penner, 1987; Bohannon & Stanowicz, 1988 and Moore, Furrow, Boyd & Chiasson, 1990. How, or if, such differential response patterns could provide useful information for the child is still the subject of continuing debate (Morgan & Travis, 1989; Marcus, 1993) but the evidence suggests, at least, that they exist. Overall, children's WFUs tend to be followed by different types of responses from their IFUs. A summary of the earlier research findings is shown in Table 6.1; some of the terms used for these response categories are explained further in the section dealing with our own coding scheme.

Table 6.1 Summary of differential responses to children's utterances from earlier research studies

	Grammatical (WFUs)	Ungrammatical (IFUs)
Hirsh-Pasek, Treiman & Schneiderman (1984)	Not repeated	Repeated
Demetras, Post & Snow (1986) reply	Move on Exact repetition	Clarification Q Extended/contracted
Bohannon & Stanowicz (1988)	Exact repetition Exact repetition	Recast repetition Recast repetition
Penner (1987)	Topic extension	Expansion
Moore, Furrow Boyd & Chiasson (1990)	Exact repetition Move ons	Clarification Q Expansions Recasts

This study is concerned with the case of profoundly deaf children learning to speak, who typically have particular difficulties in acquiring grammar. Deaf children's experience of spoken langugage is seriously impoverished (Swisher, 1989) and this may be the case for at least two reasons. First, crucial linguistic items may be difficult or even impossible to perceive, because of their lack of salience. Plural and past tense markers, verbal auxiliaries and modals, prepositions and determiners are all frequently unstressed and are generally much more difficult to hear than content words — so it may be particularly difficult to extract the necessary information from spoken language (de Villiers & de Villiers, 1994). Secondly, interaction patterns may differ from the typical hearing situation and may offer even less potentially useful feedback. The speech of young deaf children may be relatively unintelligible and so their mothers may fail to expand their children's utterances because of difficulties in understanding them (Lyon, 1985), thus providing less negative feedback than is available to normally hearing children. The aim of this study was to consider whether deaf children could potentially experience similar types of differential response to IFUs and WFUs.

The Coding Scheme

The coding schemes for maternal and child utterances were based on, and adapted from, the categories in earlier studies. All child multi-word utterances were classified into three categories:

Well-formed utterances (WFUs)
Ill-formed utterances (IFUs)
Phonologically unclear utterances (PUs)

The distinction between WFUs and IFUs is not always obvious or straightforward. Child utterances can be immature or incorrect for various reasons, some of which may involve vocabulary or the appropriacy of an utterance in context. Here, grammatical criteria were used (omission of obligatory morphemes, wrong word order, etc.) to judge whether utterances were WF or IF. Formally correct sentences were classed as WF even if inappropriate or including wrong vocabulary. In practice, errors rarely fell into this category. Some utterances would have been acceptably elliptical in conversational discourse in adult speech, e.g. *next one* rather than *the next one*. In this study, instances such as this were judged WF.

The maternal language coding scheme was as follows:

(1) *Repetition (REP)*

- exact repetition
- partial repetition without change or addition
- repetition with intonation pattern implying a question
- repetition exact except for deictic adjustments.

(2) *Clarification Question (CQ)*

Any question which a) repeats part of preceding utterance, b) does not request new information and c) is not an exact repetition apart from intonation.

(3) *Expansion (EXP)*

Repetition that expands or diverges from preceding child utterance without providing corrective information.

(4) *Recast (REC)*

Repetition that diverges from preceding child utterance in such a way as to provide corrective information.

(5) *Move-on (M-O)*

Any verbal response which is neither wholly nor partly a repetition.

(6) *No response (NR)*

Some classification decisions were problematic. For example, it might seem logical to treat questions that are exact repetitions except for intonation as clarification questions. Demetras *et al.* do so, and find clarification questions are associated with IFUs. However, Bohannon & Stanowicz treat questions which are exact repetitions as a separate category, 'exact questions', and find they are used similarly to exact repetitions, mostly in response to WFUs. Here, such questions were treated as repetitions.

Of the studies mentioned, only Moore *et al.* had a special category (recasts) for responses that provided corrective information, and they collapsed it with expansions because they got so few examples. There is a methodological objection to treating recasts as a separate category; it is logically impossible for a response which supplies corrective information to be a response to a WFU. However, the availability of corrective information is crucial to some forms of the negative feedback argument, so the decision was made to identify recasts separately in the first instance.

The term *move-on* is defined negatively by both Demetras *et al.* and Moore *et al.* as the absence of repetition, which has been followed here as appropriate to the focus of the study — however, the potentially misleading use of the term *move-on* as a discourse classification should be borne in mind.

Subjects and Data

The subjects were three profoundly deaf children who had been attending speech and hearing clinics at the University of Manchester and were being brought up within an auditory/oral approach. They were two boys, FD and HB, and one girl, KL, all within the normal intelligence range, with no additional handicaps. All had hearing losses in excess of 90 dB. They had been attending the clinic at regular three-monthly intervals since diagnosis of their hearing loss. Each visit included a short videorecorded play session with mother and child in a specially designed clinic. Although mothers and children had attended often enough to be reasonably at home in the clinic, the possible effects of the clinic environment cannot be ruled out. Here, the language level of the children was considered rather than their age, and accordingly, videotapes were scanned for multi-word utterances. Three suitable ten-minute clips for each child were identified and transcribed (because of small numbers, data from the three occasions were collapsed for each child) as can be seen in Table 6.2.

Results

The data tables in this section show the pattern of responses summed across all three tapes for each child individually and then overall. Raw scores are given rather than percentages as numbers were small (see Tables 6.3–6.6).

The most likely response to HB's WFUs was to repeat them (although the full range of other responses also occurred, see Table 6.3). To IFUs, almost half of the responses were recasts, and a further fifth were clarification requests. With respect to the unclear utterances, the responses were distributed over all categories.

FD's mother used no clarification questions at all. There were very few recasts; indeed, in this case no identifiable pattern which could provide differential feedback emerges (see Table 6.4).

Table 6.2 Summary of data

		Child utterances total	Multi-Word child utterances	Maternal utterances
FD1	1;9	88	14	253
FD2	2;3	92	16	213
FD3	2;6	80	12	225
HB1	2;10	127	8	253
HB2	3;0	56	7	N.A.
HB3	3;7	120	54	224
KL1	2;11	126	28	340
KL2	3;3	85	29	325
KL3	3;10	178	44	370

(*Note:* HB 2 included some interaction with the subject's baby sister.)

Table 6.3 HB: summary of maternal responses to child utterances

	REP	CQ	EXP	REC	M-O	NR	TOTALS
WFUs	8	1	5	1	3	3	21
IFUs	2	7	4	17	4	2	36
PUs	4	6	5	2	7	4	28
TOTALS	14	14	14	20	14	9	85

Table 6.4 FD: summary of maternal responses to child utterances

	REP	CQ	EXP	REC	M-O	NR	TOTALS
WFUs	6	–	6	–	6	4	22
IFUs	3	–	1	2	7	1	14
PUs	1	–	2	–	4	1	8
TOTALS	10	–	9	2	17	6	44

Table 6.5   KL: summary of maternal responses to child utterances

	REP	CQ	EXP	REC	M-O	NR	TOTALS
WFUs	9	4	15	–	18	2	48
IFUs	14	5	7	14	6	2	48
PUs	1	2	3	–	4	–	10
TOTALS	24	11	25	14	28	4	106

With KL, a different pattern again emerges (see Table 6.5). WFUs are typically responded to by either an expansion or a move-on; these two categories combined account for nearly three-quarters of answers to well-formed. IFUs attract all kinds of responses, but most typically repetitions and recasts.

Considering all three child–mother pairs, one noticeable pattern is that the NR category is tiny; that is, all three mothers almost invariably made some response to child utterances even if they were phonologically unclear. However, FD's mother did not respond to 6 out of 44 of the multi-word utterances in our data, whereas for KL's mother, only 4 out of 106 utterances remained unanswered. (It must be remembered that these data excluded SWUs (single word utterances), so no firm statement can be made about how *generally* responsive the mothers were.)

Both HB's and KL's mothers frequently recast IFUs, but FD's mother rarely did so. Given that it has been suggested that recasts may facilitate grammatical development (Baker & Nelson, 1984; Farrar, 1990; Farrar, 1992), it might be suggested that at least on these clinic occasions, FD's mother was less well-tuned and provided less helpful feedback than did the other two mothers. However, the possibility arises than FD's IFUs were for some reason less easy to recast than those of the others. Moreover, though there is some evidence that recasts tend to be helpful, we do not know if this is true in all circumstances or, if not, in which.

Table 6.6   Summary of maternal responses: totals for all three children

	REP	CQ	EXP	REC	M-O	NR	TOTALS
WFUs	23	5	26	1	27	9	91
IFUs	19	12	12	33	17	5	98
PUs	6	8	10	2	15	5	46
TOTALS	48	25	48	36	59	19	235

Overall, child IFUs were much more likely to be followed by clarification questions and recasts than WFUs were, and less likely to be followed by move-ons (see Table 6.6).

Children at this stage of language development produce few multi-word utterances, and consequently, when the responses have been divided into several categories, numbers are very small. For robust results to emerge, studies need to be based on extensive data collection. Our coding system was designed to provide results which could be compared to earlier studies with hearing children. It is not without problems, and ideally, any future study should also include more detailed analyses of individual utterances and response patterns. However, an interesting response pattern could be observed. First, child WFUs and IFUs attract different response patterns from the mothers of at least some hearing impaired children, and second, some differences between mothers emerge, even from a sample of only three. The fact that some clear patterns have emerged point to the likely value of future investigations along these lines.

References

Baker, N. D. and Nelson, K. E. (1984) Recasting and related conversational techniques for triggering syntactic advances by young children. *First Language*.

Bohannon, J. N. and Stanowicz, L. (1988) The issue of negative evidence: Adult responses to children's language errors. *Developmental Psychology* 24, 684–89.

Brown, R. (1973) *A First Language*. Cambridge, MA: Harvard University Press.

Brown, R. and Hanlon, C. (1970) Derivational complexity and order of acquisition in child speech. In J. R. Hayes (ed.) *Cognition and the Development of Language*. New York: Wiley.

De Villiers, J.D. and de Villiers, P.A. (1994) The central problem of functional categories in the English syntax of oral deaf children. In H. Tager-Flusberg (ed.) *Constraints on Language Acquisition: Studies of Atypical Children*. Hillsdale, NJ: Lawrence Erlbaum Associates.

Demetras, M., Post, K. and Snow, C. (1986) Feedback to first-language learners. *Journal of Child Language* 13, 275–92.

Farrar, M. (1992) Negative evidence and grammatical morpheme acquisition. *Developmental Psychology* 28, 91–9.

Farrar, M. J. (1990) Discourse and the acquisition of grammatical morphemes. *Journal of Child Language* 17, 607–24.

Hirsh-Pasek, K., Treiman, R. and Schneiderman, M. (1984) Brown & Hanlon revisited: mother's sensitivity to ungrammatical forms. *Journal of Child Language* 11, 81–8.

Lyon, M. (1985) The verbal interaction of mothers and their pre-school hearing-impaired children: A preliminary investigation. *Journal of the British Association of Teachers of the Deaf* 9, 119–29.

Marcus, G.F. (1993) Negative evidence in language acquisition. *Cognition* 46, 53–85.

Moore, C., Furrow, D., Boyd, G. and Chiasson, L. (1990) Differential feedback to children's language errors: Effects of and on developmental level. Paper presented at Budapest, IASCL Conference, July, 1990.

Morgan, J.L. and Travis, L.L. (1989) Limits on negative information in language input. *Journal of Child Language* 16, 531–52.

Penner, S. G. (1987) Parental responses to grammatical and ungrammatical child utterances. *Child Development* 58, 376–84.

Swisher, M.V. (1989) The language-learning situation of deaf students. *TESOL Quarterly* 23, 239–57.

7 Negation and Truncated Structures

CORNELIA HAMANN

Verb-raising and Negation in Acquisition

In recent acquisition research, the position of the verb relative to the negation particle has been used to argue for the early existence of verb movement in children's grammars of French, German, and other languages. The argument is based on the distribution of finite and non-finite verbs with respect to the negative particle. Pierce (1989) demonstrated that French children place the non-finite verb after the negative particle *pas*, but place finite verbs before this particle at a surprisingly early age and almost without errors, cf. (1a,1b) and Table 7.1 for the distribution of negation over three children covering an age span of 1;8–2;6.

(1a) pas tomber bébé   (b) veux pas lolo   Nathalie 2;0.1
     not fall baby   want not water

Table 7.1 Finite and non-finite verbs with negation (Pierce, 1989)

	–Fin	+Fin
pas Verb	77	11
Verb pas	2	185
total	79	196

Similar results have been obtained by Verrips and Weissenborn (1989) for German and French and have been corroborated by Hamann (1993a). The conclusion is that in French and German finite verbs raise across negation and infinitives remain below, or in other words, finite verbs raise to the inflectional phrase (IP), while infinitives stay in the verbal phrase (VP). The implication of these findings is that children at the age of around two years have the finiteness distinction and a functional projection for the finite verb to raise to, i.e. they already have IP at least. However, there are two questions to be asked in the context of recent linguistic theory.

Given the introduction of the negative phrase (NegP) as a functional category by Pollock (1989), and given the acquisition of (some) functional categories at that age, it seems to follow from the above that negative particles across which the verb can raise must be specifiers, as is clear for French *pas*. For German *nicht* and English *not* there is a lively debate, however, with regard to their status as negative head or specifier. If acquisition literature assumes that these particles are heads at least in child language, it has to answer the question how the verb can raise across another head unless there is cliticization, and how a reclassification comes about if the particle in question is a specifier in the adult language. If a reclassification takes place, we face the problem of discontinuity. Therefore the first question to be answered is whether anything is gained by assuming that the negative particle is a head in the child grammar of German.

The second problem concerns the child's truncation option (Rizzi, 1993; 1994). Originally conceived to explain the optionality of infinitives and null subjects at a certain stage in acquisition, the theory proposes that the child can truncate structure at any point in the tree. The child projects only as much structure as is necessary to accommodate the morphological material present in the phrase, in accordance with the Minimalize Structure Constraint proposed by Grimshaw (1993). Thus the child does not project further than VP for an infinitival clause, but can in the next instance use an inflected verb which has been raised to IP.

Taken together with the assumption of a universally given order of projections, this hypothesis makes very precise co-occurrence predictions. If the NegP selects the temporal phrase (TP), then it follows that the use of negation will activate finiteness and thus exclude the sequence *Neg Infinitive* in principle. So the second question is, whether the occurrence of negation with infinitives is robust or not. If it is rare across languages then Rizzi's proposal is proved correct. If it is robust in some languages, but rare in others, then the order of projections cannot be universal, or negation in the particular language is an adverb. If the phenomenon is robust in languages where it is well established that NegP is above TP, then Rizzi's proposal needs revision.

The NegP and the Neg Criterion

Based on Pollock (1989) and other work, it has generally been accepted that the clause structure of English and of French contains a functional projection NegP. In French this functional projection is headed by *ne* which has to co-occur with another negative constituent (2), and a dependency relation between the negative head and the negative constituents has been observed. The head not only requires the presence of another negative projection (XP), but empty category principle (ECP) effects surface in (3a,3b). In parallel to work on Wh-questions (Rizzi, 1991) this dependency has been explained by postulating a well formedness condition at the level of logical form (LF), (cf. Haegeman & Zanuttini, 1991 and Haegeman, 1991). This condition, which determines the distribution of negative elements, is formulated as the Neg Criterion.

(2)   Jean ne viendra *(pas/jamais)

         J.   ne come(fut) not/never

(3a)   Je n'exige que tu voies personne

         I ne insist that you see nobody

(3b)   Je n'exige que personne vienne (*personne* can only have narrow scope)

         I ne insist that nobody come

Neg Criterion

i.   A NEG-operator must be in a Spec-head configuration with an X^0 [NEG].

ii.   An X^0 [NEG] must be in a Spec-head configuration with a NEG-operator.

The Neg Criterion applies as late as LF in French, which will immediately account for the ECP effects in (3a and b). In these examples LF movement of *personne* is due to the Neg Criterion. In other languages, the Neg Criterion applies at the level of surface-structure. West Flemish (WF) is a case in point as argued in Haegeman (in prep). WF also shows the phenomenon of negative concord, i.e. the occurrence of two negative expressions leads to a simple negation reading. In such constructions, not just one, but all negative constituents must be in a specifier-head relation with the negative head *en* at S-structure. This is achieved by either moving a negative consitutent to SpecNegP, or by moving it to the specifier of a higher functional projection which thus becomes an extended projection of the NegP. Thus also an 'extended specifier head relation with *en*' can satisfy the Neg Criterion.

The possibility to form an extended projection of the NegP will be relevant for the account of the acquisition sequence in German presented here in so far as German shows many parallels to WF even if it does not have a two-partite negation. As Hamann (1993a, b) show, German patterns with WF in that the Neg Criterion has to be satisfied at S-structure — something which might be related to the properties of scrambling in these languages. Such a parallel to WF certainly presupposes the existence of a NegP or a Polarity phrase (PolP) in

German. If we assume a PolP, then the negative particle will colour it negatively and make it into a NegP.

Negation in German and the Head/Specifier Problem

Negation, verb movement and acquisition — a dilemma?

Acquisition research, with the exception of Deprez and Pierce (1990, 1993), assumes that *nicht* is the head of a NegP or that there is an early misclassification as a head (cf. Clahsen, 1988; Verrips & Weissenborn, 1989; Penner, Tracy & Weissenborn, 1994). Such an analysis tries to capture some phenomena of early negation. It can explain examples like 4(a) where the negative particle seems to cliticise to the modal or auxiliary. Such a cliticlike affinity of the verb and the negative particle can also explain examples like (4b and c) where the object has not scrambled in child language but scrambles across negation in adult language.

(4a) will nich, mag nich, kann nich etc.   as found in all corpora.

 want not, like not, cannot

(4b) macht nich aua   Simone 1;10.3 (Verrips & Weissenborn, 1989)

 makes not ouch

(4c) baby nich nuckel habe Simone 2;0.0   (Verrips &Weissenborn, 1989)

 baby not pacifier have

The contrast in verb placement of (4b) and (4c) is then used to argue for verb movement in parallel to the arguments for French. This gets us into the dilemma sketched above. Either we assume head movement across another head, or we assume that the negative particle has cliticised and moves along with the verb, in which case we cannot honestly say anything about positions and raising.

Nicht is not a head in adult Standard German

For adult German Bayer (1990) investigated the phenomenon of Bavarian negative concord and argued that *nicht* is a head — while Grewendorf (1990) and Haegeman (in prep.) claim that *nicht* is a specifier. Bayer's analysis cannot be appplied to Standard German, however, because there is no Neg-Verb complex: 1) *nicht* does not cliticise or move along with the verb (5b), and 2) material can intervene between *nicht* and the verb (6a to 6c).

(5a) Warum hast du das nicht gemacht?

 why   has you that not done

(5b) *Warum nicht-hast/hast-nicht du das gemacht?

 why   not-have/have-not you that done

(6a) daß Peter wahrscheinlich nicht nach Hause geht

      that P probably   not to   home goes

(6b) daß Peter wahrscheinlich nicht darüber sprechen will

      that P probably   not thereof talk   wants

(6c) daß Fiete da wahrscheinlich nich über sprechen will (Northern variety)

      that F there probably   not of talk   wants

We conclude that parallel to the WF specifier *nie*, German *nicht* does not incorporate and does not adjoin to other heads. So it is certainly not a clitic, and most likely not a head. If it were a head, it would be a free morpheme and as such should block verb movement — which it doesn't. There are two more facts arguing against a head status of German negation. There is the historical development, showing that *niht*, originally the enforcement of the Middle High German head *en/ne/ni*, can now stand alone. Additionally, there is the fact that Standard High German does not have negative concord, while languages with strong negative heads usually do. Let us thus conclude that *nicht* is not a head.

The Acquisition of *Nicht*

Early (mis)-classification as a head?

Even if *nicht* is not a head in adult German, there remains the possibility that there is an early misclassification. The arguments for such a misclassification would be drawn from (4a) or the object 'left behind' in (4b) and (4c).

Such an analysis is attractive, however, also for another reason. If *nicht* is initially a head, then the use of a NegP/PolP can be taken as the 'Beginning of Syntax'. This has been suggested by Penner, Tracy and Weissenborn (1994) stemming from their observation that either the subject or the object moves in early *auch-* or negated structures, but never both. Their explanation goes as follows. At 18–20 months, the child only has a very general Affect Criterion, which requires just an A'-position and a Spec-head relation of the relevant material. This A'-position is created by the presence of the heads *nicht* or *auch* and precisely the 'Ur'-form of the criteria, the requirement of a Spec-head relation.

Now one might ask why the child should place a scope bearing element in a head position and not in an operator position from the beginning. Moreover, the Neg Criterion can be seen as a special instance of feature checking. Thus it is not clear at all why the child should know about this mechanism in the case of the finiteness feature but be unable to give it a negative instantiation once the feature carrying negative morpheme is used. Thus it is not clear how an Ur-form of feature checking can exist, without knowledge of its particular instantiations — once the morpheme is present. So the story needs careful checking as to its validity.

It is clear that it cannot work if the Neg Criterion is operative, because in that case only negative material can occur as specifier and we expect utterances very similar to (1) or we even expect a phase of negative concord. But negative concord cannot be said to exist in child German as the data in Hamann (1993a) show.

Nicht as a specifier in child language

There is another possibility short of saying that *nicht* is a specifier from early on. This involves a phenomenon which Penner, Tracy and Weissenborn (1994) call freezing. They observe that in positive utterances, the child uses inflection and raises the verb while in early negative utterances and *auch*-structures, the child uses only infinitives and scrambles only the object or the subject, but not both. The explanation which comes to mind is that the child is not sure about the categorization yet and thus deliberately picks a form of the verb which does not have to be moved. This implies that the 'V_{finite} Neg'-patterns as in (7) will appear only after the child has decided that *nicht* is in a specifier position and does not block verb movement.

(7) Annette will nich   Andreas 2;1   Childes, Wagner

    A.   wants not

There are four problems with the freezing idea. First, we have the triggering problem in its usual form. Second, the phenomenon of unscrambled objects persists into a phase where negation is definitely used in finite contexts and so must be a specifier. Third, the phenomenon of freezing, i.e. an exclusive use of negation with infinitives in an early phase is not at all evident from the known data (cf. Verrips & Weissenborn, 1989). Fourth, reclassification is said to be achieved with the acquisition of *kein*, but this occurs surprisingly early for some children (Katrin, 1;5, McWhinney & Snow, 1985) and moreover some objects remain unscrambled even after the firm acquisition of *kein*. See Hamann (in prep) for more details and examples.

Such unscrambled objects thus clearly need an explanation which does not appeal to the head status of *nicht*. This might take the form of a case story or might involve focusing facts or come down to constituent negation. As to an explanation of the type of utterance exemplified in (4a), these clearly involve cliticisation on the phonological level, but need not invoke any head status of *nicht*, just as in the case of French subject clitics where an XP is cliticised to I^0.

As there is nothing to be gained in the assumption of a head

classification for an early phase of negation, while the problems of such
an approach are manifold, let us propose a scenario where *nicht* is a
specifier from the beginning. Assuming that objects remain unscrambled
for lack of case and case morphology (Eisenbeiß, 1994), the only fact to be
explained now is the one-element-only-scrambling. This can be taken care
of in the manner of Penner, Tracy and Weissenborn (1994), but with the
help of the Neg Criterion and the early acquisition of *kein*. With the
acquisition of *kein* the extended NegP becomes available, providing one
and only one additional position. This can be an object-agreement phrase
(AgrOP), but may be neutral as to an accusative case feature in the
beginning.

The analysis of infinitive examples where the subject has moved across
Neg (4c) requires an intermediate projection in any case. Let us call it IntP,
for intermediate projection. Such an analysis predicts a short phase of
moving one-element-only, but it does not strictly predict freezing. This is
as it should be because the known data do not corroborate freezing in
early German *nicht*-constructions. The scramble-one-only phenomenon
will surface only in infinitives, as observed by Penner, Tracy and
Weissenborn (1994) because for inflected verbs SpecIP provides a second
landing site.

(8) IP

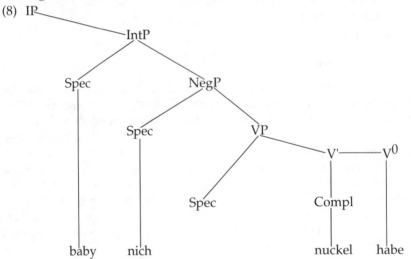

Negation and Infinitives

The truncation option and the order of projections

Our discussion so far has taken for granted that negation does occur
with infinitives in early phases in German. With the recent theory of
truncated structures as proposed in Rizzi (1993, 1994), negation should
not occur with infinitives at all.

The theory was devised to account for optional infinitives, especially the observation that optional infinitives do not occur in Wh-questions. Wexler (1994) explained this by saying that children do not have tense at an early age or have underspecified tense features. Rizzi (1994) captures the impression that the complementiser phrase (CP) cannot be involved in these optional infinitives by postulating that the adult axiom *CP = root* is not yet operative for children. Therefore children can *truncate* at any place in the tree, in the case of infinitives at VP-level or above AgrOP. If a projection higher than TP is involved, the tense morpheme necessarily has to be bound, so infinitives cannot occur. Thus with a tree as assumed by Belletti (1990) in (9), it follows that negation cannot occur with infinitives.

(9)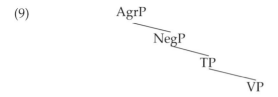

If the NegP is lower than TP in the language, i.e. the order of projections has to be parametrized, or if there is a special sort of adverbial negation associated with infinitives as seems to be the case for Dutch (see Hoekstra & Jordens, 1991: V_{fin} *niet* but *nee* V_{-fin}), or if Neg is an adverb in that phase (or in that language), then negation can occur with infinitives. If we find infinitives with negation across languages or in languages were the order of projections is as in (9) for theoretical reasons, then Rizzi's assumption needs revision.

A first look at German data shows that negation is rarer with infinitives than with finite constructions. For the child Andreas we find an equal percentage of infinitives in positive and negative utterances, however.

Table 7.2 Distribution of infinitives in verbal utterances in German

		Katrin, 1;5			Andreas, 2;1	
	Total	−Fin	+Fin	Total	−Fin	+Fin
all verbal utt	415	167 40%	248 60%	785	218 28%	567 72%
pos verb utt	403	167 42%	236 58%	729	204 28%	525 72%
neg verbal utt	12	0	12	56	14 25%	42 75%

Nicht as an adverb, Topicalizing *Nicht*

This result fits together with a set of data found in German, which point to an adverb use of *nicht*. This is the topicalization of the negative particle in child language.

(10a) Nicht will ich das Schwarze   Elena 3;5   Hamann diary notes

        not   want I the black

(10b) fels noch nich is er putt   Daniel 2;9   Childes, Clahsen

        rock not yet is he broken

(10c) ni kommt zurück   Mathias 2;10 Childes, Clahsen

        not comes back

(10d) nich geht er putt   Mathias 2;10 Childes, Clahsen

        not goes he broken

(10e) nich fährt   Mathias 2;10 Childes, Clahsen

        not drives

The fact that Swedish *inte*, Norwegian *ikke* can be topicalized, but Danish *ikke* and German *nicht* cannot, indicates a solution. Let us assume that in adult German *nicht* as SpecNeg is base inserted, the Neg Criterion is satisfied right there and thus no further movement is possible for economy reasons. Then it follows that child German, Swedish, and Norwegian treat negation as an adverb (just as *gar nicht* must be an adverb and can be topicalized in German). This is in accordance with other researchers' assumptions (cf. Wode, 1977 and Clahsen, 1988 for German, Hoekstra & Jordens, 1991 for Dutch, and Radford, 1990 for English).

Such an adverb classification does not exclude the possibility of having a low NegP in German because it makes it possible for the negative particle to occupy the specifier of the PolP and colour it negatively. But it would also explain the external negation phase, and the many occurrences of constituent negation and so the unscrambled objects. The negative adverb would occupy whatever specifier is necessary to acquire the envisaged scope relation.

Attractive though this analysis is, there is a problem: Particle verbs tend to occur in the infinitive in this phase of development, i.e. they distort the count. If we deduct them, we are left with almost no occurrences of negation with infinitive.

Table 7.3 Distribution of infinitives in verbal utterances without particle verbs

		Katrin, 1;5			Andreas, 2;1	
	Total	−Fin	+Fin	Total	−Fin	+Fin
all verbal	362	131	231	646	101	545
utt		36%	64%		16%	84%
pos verb	350	131	219	603	97	506
utt		37%	63%		16%	84%
neg verbal	12	0	12	43	4	39
utt					9%	91%

Table 7.4

Julia, 1;11–2;5	verbal utterances			verbal utterances without particle verbs		
	Total	Inf	+Fin	Total	Inf	+Fin
all utt	193	93 (48.2%)	100 (51.8%)	143	44 (30.8%)	99 (69.2%)
pos utt	170	88 (51.8%)	82 (48.2%)	121	41 (34.7%)	79 (65.3%)
neg utt	25	5 (20%)	20 (80%)	22	2 (9.1%)	20 (90.9%)

Four cases of negative infinitives remain in the Andreas corpus. One of these is a normal elliptical answer to a question and one is the normal adult jussive use as in *nicht anfassen, nicht loslassen, nicht hinauslehnen*. So only two cases remain and thus negation is extremely rare with infinitives if one does not count cases of particle verbs. Clahsen's Julia corpus shows the same. Negation occurs with infinitives, but without counting particle constructions, the infinitive cases are negligible. Thus we must conclude that negation might be an adverb in German, but that the issue about the order of projections remains open, as long as the particle verb issue remains open. A look at French data shows that even there the situation is not clear at all. Let us return to Pierce's results. We find that about 29% of the negative utterances found in three corpora occur in the infinitive. Even discounting the 50 cases of infinitives from Nathalie's first file, the figures (13% of infinitives in negative utterances) are in the same range as those found for German. There is one problem with this result for our purposes, however. Pierce (1989) counted non-finite constructions, which include bare participles. These behave differently from infinitives in many respects. So Friedemann (1992) did not include bare participles and arrived at a much lower figure. He reports only about 5% of infinitives in negative utterances. On the other hand, a recent count on a new corpus arrives at the higher percentage of 12% again.

Table 7.5 Distribution of *infinitives* in verbal utterances in French

all verbal utterances			negative verbal utterances		
Total	−Fin	+Fin	Total	−Fin	+Fin
Philippe 2;1–2;3, Gregoire 1;11–2;3 (Friedemann, 1992)					
?	?	?	127	6 (4.7%)	121
Augustin 2;0–2;4 (Hamann, in prep)					
302	71 (23.5%)	231	8	1 (12.2%)	7

Conclusion

Given that the statistics is not very good for Augustin, there is reason to believe that Friedemann's results corroborate Rizzi's theory. For German, we need an account of negative infinitive structures at least for particle verbs, unless we assume that the child assigns some wild structure to these constructions. If we do not assume that, we are forced to accept the particle verb constructions, i.e. the negative infinitives to a rather high percentage (25%). Thus the conclusion seems to be that NegP is lower than TP in German, which has been assumed independently of acquisition data for languages like German, Dutch and West Flemish. Therefore the order of projections cannot be universal — a conclusion also reached by Haegeman (1994) in her analysis of Dutch acquisition data.

Acknowledgements

This work was made possible by the Swiss National Fund Grant No. 11-33542.92. A version of the first part of this paper was presented during the Trieste Encounters in Cognitive Science Workshop at the International School for Advanced Studies in July 1993, organized by Ken Wexler and Luigi Rizzi. The part on truncated structures grew out of discussions held in Trieste and preliminary data were presented at the Berne conference on Scrambling and Clause Internal Rules in January 1994. I thank the participants of both conferences and especially Liliane Haegeman for many valuable suggestions.

References

Bayer, J. (1990) What Bavarian negative concord reveals about the syntactic structure of German. In J. Mascaro and M. Nespor (eds) *Grammar in Progress*. Dordrecht: Foris. pp.13–23.
Belletti, A. (1990) *Generalized Verb Movement*. Turin: Rosenberg and Sellier.
Clahsen, H. (1988) Kritische Phasen der Grammatikentwicklung. *Zeitschrift für Sprachwissenschaft* 7, pp.3–31.
Deprez, V. and Pierce A. (1990) A Crosslinguistic Study of Negation in Early Syntactic Development. BU conference 1990.

— (1993) Crosslinguistic evidence for functional projections in early grammar. In T. Hoekstra and B. Schwartz (eds). *Language Acquisition Studies in Generahve Grammar*. Amsterdam: Benjamins.

Eisenbeiβ, S. (1994) Kasus und Wortstellung im deutschen Mittelfeld. Ms, Lexlern-projekt Düsseldorf.

Friedemann, M.-A. (1992) The underlying position of external arguments in French. *Geneva Generative Papers*. 1992.

Grewendorf, G. (1990) Verb-Bewegung und Negation im Deutschen. *GAGL* 30, pp. 57–125.

Grimshaw, J. (1993) Minimal projection, heads and optimality. Draft manuscript, Rutgers University, June 1993.

Haegeman, L. (1991) Negative Concord, Negative Heads. Going romance and Beyond. OTS Working Papres, OTS-WP-TL-91-002. University of Utrecht, Trans 10, 3512 Utrecht.

— (1994) Root infinitives, tense and and truncated structures. *Geneva Generative Papers*.

— (in preparation) *The Syntax of Negation*. Cambridge: Cambridge University Press.

Haegeman, L. and Zanuttini R. (1991) Negative heads and the Neg Criterion. *The Linguistic Review* 8, pp. 233–51.

Hamann, C. (1993a) On the Acquisition of Negation in German. Working paper, ISAS, Trieste, July 1993. Ms. University of Geneva.

— (1993b) Some Scope Phenomena in German Negation. Ms. University of Geneva.

— (in prep.) Negation, Infinitives and Heads.

Hoekstra, T. and Jordens P. (1991, 1993) From Adjunct to Head. Glow, 1991. Now in T. Hoekstra and B. Schwartz (eds) *Language Acquisition Studies in Generative Grammar*. Amsterdam: Benjamins.

McWhinney, B. and Snow C. (1985) The child language data exchange system. *Journal of Child Language*, 12.

Penner, Z., Tracy R. and Weissenborn J. (1994) Scrambling in Early Developmental Stages in Standard and Swiss German. Hand-out, Berne-conference on Scrambling and Clause Internal Rules, Jan 1994.

Pierce, A. (1989) The emergence of syntax: A cross linguistic study. PhD dissertation, MIT.

Pollock, J.Y. (1989) Verb movement, universal grammar and the structure of IP. *Linguistic Inquiry* 20, 365–424.

Radford, A. (1990) *Syntactic Theory and the Acquisition of English Syntax: The Nature of Early Child Grammars of English*. Oxford: Blackwell.

— (1994) The nature of children's initial clauses. Talk held at Bangor Child Language Seminar, March 1994.

Rizzi, L. (1991) Residual Verb-Second and the WH-Criterion. *Technical Reports on Formal and Computational Linguistics*. No. 2. Geneva University.

— (1993) Some notes on linguistic theory and language development. Ms. SISSA, Trieste, July 1993.

— (1994) Some notes on linguistic theory and language development. *Geneva Generative Papers*.

Verrips, M. and Weissenborn J. (with R. Berman) (1989) Negation as a Window to the Structure of Early Child Language. Ms. Nijmegen, Max-Planck-Institute.

Wexler, K. (1994) Optional infinitives, head movement and the economy of derivations in child grammar. In D. Lightfoot and N. Hornstein, *Verb Movement*. Cambridge: Cambridge University Press.

Wode, H. (1977) Four early stages in the development of LI negation. *Journal of Child Language* 4 , pp. 87–102.

8 Verb Complementation in Language Impaired School Age Children

GABRIELLE KING

Introduction

In a research project that has just drawn to a close, Paul Fletcher and I have been looking at the spontaneous conversations of language impaired and normal children with particular reference to their use of verbs and their complements.

We started with 14 children aged between 7 and 10 defined in the usual way as having Specific Language Impairment (SLI), and 14 normal children of 3, 5 and 7 years old, matched to them by Mean Length of Utterance (MLU) in morphemes.[1]

Initial Study

Initially, we analysed their output for errors of morphosyntax, looking at obligatory contexts for the supply of bound morphemes. Here we found only one significant difference, in present tense verb agreement, where the SLI subjects omitted the 3rd person -s more frequently than their normal counterparts. When we looked analogously at obligatory contexts for the supply of verb arguments, we found a greater frequency and range of verb argument errors by SLI than LN children, but the numbers do not reach significance. In Table 8.1, a summary of the relevant figures is given.[2]

Table 8.1 Errors of verb complementation (1st subect group: 14 SLI (aged 7–10) and 14 LN (aged 3–5))

Frequency of Argument Structure Errors (SLI and LN subjects n = 28)					
Subject Group	Error Type			Verb Types Affected	
	O	S	total/all V*	O	S
SLI	23	9	32/1062 (3%)	12	8
LN	15	4	19/981 (1.9%)	4	4

(*excluding verbs with legitimate zero complementation)

Following this, we concentrated on their verb complementation where it was grammatical, where we were looking for differences in the groups' deployment of verb resources.[3]

Verb Complementation Study

First we standardised sample size by the number of lexical verbs (excluding the copula *be*) in complete and intelligible utterances. This figure was 63 verbs (fixed at the bottom end by the 3 year old with the lowest MLU), and our subject groups went down to 11 from 14 as a consequence (details of the subjects' ages and MLU in morphemes can be seen in appendix 1). We developed a classification of complement-realization that resulted in 8 categories as seen in Table 8.2.

Table 8.2 Verb complementation categories

Lexical verb +	
O	no internal argument (complement)
NP	(direct) object
CLMCP	clausal (direct object) complement (e.g. *I don't know **why it's funny***)
PP	prepositional phrase or other adverbial functioning as oblique argument (e.g. *he's walking **to baby shop***)
NPPP	object and prepositional phrase (as above) (e.g. *I put **that there***)
NPNP	goal NP and direct object NP ('double object' datives, e.g. *give **us some hard ones***)
NP-to-NP	direct object NP and to followed by goal NP (prepositional dative: e.g. *I want to do **some to you***)
NPXP	small clause complements (e.g. *I not heard **horses talk**, let **that out***)

These categories are mostly unambiguous from this table. We should make it very clear that we were classifying those elements that were realized, and not those which would be required by the verb in question. So for instance, the 0 category will apply to verbs known as intransitives, but just as importantly, to many other 'transitive' verbs where their characteristic direct object requirement may be waived (examples of this kind of zero-complementation can be seen in appendix 2). The other category which needs a little explanation is the last, the NPXP category. This is a shorthand for what are sometimes called 'small clauses', like *horses talk* or *that out* following the verbs *hear* and *let* in Table 8.2. They are called small clauses because the relation of the NP object to what follows it is like that of a subject to its predicate.[4]

We should also make clear our choice of terminology. Many locative or goal elements, realized as an adverb or a prepositional phrase (and labelled PP above), would be argued to be adjuncts and not arguments of the verb. Our use of the term 'complement' for all these elements blurs the distinction between arguments of the verb and adjuncts to the verb phrase. This decision was motivated both by our methodology (in that we needed to label whatever the children chose to combine with particular lexical verbs) but also because we felt the lack of any workable tests distinguishing the one from the other.

Results

When this classification of verb complements was applied to each child's 63-verb sample, the results were as seen in Table 8.3.

Table 8.3 Complementation analysis (2nd subject group: 11 SLI, 11 LN (3, 5 and 7 year olds)

Subject Group	0	NP	CLCMP	PP	NPPP	NPNP	NPtoNP	NPXP	n
SLI	95	282	53	145	95	3	1	19	693
LN	67	222	48	215	135	3	0	3	693

From this Table it appeared that SLI subjects might be using many more verbs with zero complementation and fewer verbs with the NPPP complementation than the language normals. But when we looked instead at each individual SLI child and their LN matched pair, it was clear that these differences only held for a subgroup of 5, whereas for the remaining 6, there was no systematic distinction between the pairs of language impaired and normal children (see Table 8.4). The SLI children in this subgroup have, broadly, the lowest MLU scores and all have some comprehension delay (from 1 to 33 months).

Table 8.4 Subgroup of 5 pairs (3rd group: 5 SLI, 5 LN)

Subject Group	0	NP	CLCMP	PP	NPPP	NPNP	NPtoNP	NPXP	n
SLI	62	108	23	66	46	2	0	8	315
LN	20	93	17	73	111	0	0	1	315

We looked into various possible explanations for these 2 differences in complementation, and anything that might connect them. We know that lexical choice is not at the root of the difference, because the difference remains if we only looked at verbs common to both groups.

Then we looked at only those verbs which participate in the CAUSATIVE/INCHOATIVE alternation. This alternation refers to verbs like *move* which in its inchoative form is used without a direct object, with the subject carrying the thematic role of theme or patient of the action, for example in *it moved quietly*. If a direct object appears, then the subject is the agent of the action, as in *I moved it quietly*. These ten subjects used a total of 16 verb types which enter into the causative/inchoative alternation, and their uses of the 2 alternants were see in Table 8.5 (examples may be seen in Appendix 2).

Table 8.5 Complementation of causative/inchoative alternating verbs (Raw scores for a subgroup of 5 pairs of children)

		Inchoative Complements	Causative Complements			
Subjects	0	PP	NP	NPPP	total types	total tokens
SLI	8	6	6	2	14	22
LN	2	4	13	15	12	34

Table 8.5a Causative/inchoative percentage use (subgroup of 5 pairs of children)

Subject	Inchoative use	Causative use
SLI	64	36
LN	18	82

It is clear then, that the SLI children much prefer the inchoative, while the LN children prefer the causative forms. This is the strongest indication we have found of a connection between cells with significant differences in Table 8.4, that is, the high zero and low NPPP complementation by SLI, and the converse from the LN children. So it seems that a preference for the inchoative among these particular SLI children is involving them in the use of more verbs with no complement at all, and much less use of an NP and a PP complement, while the reverse follows from the normal children's preference for the causative alternation.

Table 8.6 Non-alternating verbs (%) (subgroup of 5 pairs of children)

Subject Group	0	NP	CLCMP	PP	NPPP	NPNP	NPtoNP	NPXP
SLI	18	36	8	21	15	0	0	2
LN	6	29	6	25	34	0	0	0

Lastly, in Table 8.6 we can see what is left when these alternating verbs are removed from Table 8.4's figures. The differences in the zero and the NPPP columns still hold. So whatever we might conclude as to these 5 SLI children's thematic preferences, it does not in any case tell the whole story. When we look at non-alternating verbs we find that the SLI children still delete more direct objects, where that is an option (e.g. with *bite* or *win*) and similarly use fewer PP-Type complements with verbs of motion or location like *go* or *walk* (examples of utterances from our data which show this kind of difference are given in Appendix 2).

In the NPPP category, the difference is largely explained by the much more frequent use of *put* and *take* with the NPPP complement by the language normal subgroup. It still appears that instead of using these verbs with an NP and a PP complement, the impaired group are selecting other verbs and using a single complement with them.

Conclusions

So we seem to have three types of evidence pointing to a reduction strategy by these 5 language impaired children. One is their choice, with verbs entering into the causative/inchoative alternation, for the inchoative alternant. The second is their greater omission of single verb complements (objects or prepositional phrases) where these are not obligatory. Both these kinds of reduction result in zero complementation of the verb. The third type of evidence from the subgroup of language impaired children was their less frequent use of verbs taking the double arguments of NP+PP.

But these three strands of evidence have to be taken alongside the indication we found that these children's syntactic ability is not depressed relative to their normal counterparts, recalling their greater use of clausal and small-clausal complements (see Table 8.4). In addition, we drew attention to the lack of evidence that these 5 language impaired children had any gaps in their lexicons where verbs or their argument structures were concerned. So at least for the particular type of impairment found in these children, our results may be viewed as consistent with explanations of Specific Language Impairment as a capacity limitation rather than a representational deficit.

Notes

1. The use of MLU as a measure of language age has been upheld up to the value of 6, or around 5 years of age for normal children, in a large sample study by Miller and Chapman (1981).
2. Details of both morphosyntactic and verb-complementation errors can be found in King and Fletcher (1993).
3. We found no evidence that the SLI children's verb vocabulary was limited relative to their normal peers.
4. The term 'small clause' is still controversial. Its central assumption is that at its head is a single constituent. One alternative analysis, favoured here, is to treat these as 'resultative predicates', involving 2 constituents. Another alternative for some cases (such as *let that out*) is to treat them as direct-object+particle combinations, rather like our NP+PP complement. For a discussion, see Radford (1988: 324ff).

Appendix 1

Subject details: chronological ages and MLU (in morphemes) of matched subjects.

c.a = chronological age in years and months

	SLI	*c.a.*	*MLU*	*LN*	*c.a.*	*MLU*
1	AM	7;3	3.43	GA	3;3	3.49
2	SHE	7;10	3.81	LE	3;1	3.63
3	DAV	8;1	3.93	ST	5;2	3.66
4	PE	7;9	4.04	KSK	3;3	4.32
5	DAM	7;0	4.43	KRS	3;0	4.48
6	ZA	8;3	4.51	LS	7;1	4.87
7	JUL	9;1	4.66	JE	3;0	4.50
8	SEA	9;11	5.07	CL	7;0	5.18
9	DA	7;7	5.21	KE	6;9	5.32
10	CH	8;7	5.53	RA	5;0	5.34
11	AN	9;8	6.00	KA	7;1	5.79

Appendix 2

Examples of Verb uses showing contrasting complementations of identical lexical verbs.

(i)   *causative/inchoative alternations*

SLI children:
SLI/DAV: C when I'm very very good I can move [0].
SLI/AM: C and it's x sticking there [PP].
SLI/PE: C I let them get out [PP].

Language Normal children:
LN/ST: C I'm moving some of them [NP].
LN/GA: C I stick this on here [NPPP].
LN/LE: C I get the horsie off [NPPP].

(ii)   *Non-alternating: SLI zero complementing, LN object-complementing*

SLI children:
SLI/DAV: C some dogs bite [0].
SLI/AM: C he just looking at the mother horsie eating [NPXP].
SLI/ZA: C {F} I (do) forgotten [0] now.

Language Normal children:
LN/LS: C {F} I forgot the chairs [NP].
LN/KSK: C eating some dinner [NP].
           C it's not going to bite me [NP].
LN/KSK: C that's a dog.
           C kiss him [NP].

(iii)   *Non-alternating: SLI zero-complementing, LN PP-complementing*

SLI Children:
SLI/DAV: C and it is gonna come [0] tomorrow.
SLI/PE: E where does the wardrobe go?
           C here.
           E outside the house?
           C it's running [0] .
           ......
           C and she were walking [0] .
SLI/AM: C you (want to look at) want to look [0].
SLI/AM: C and he can walk [0].

Language Normals:

LN/ST: C that's coming off [PP].

.....

C she's [AUX] look[V]/ing backwards [PP] there.

LN/GA: C you come to my house [PP].

LN/KSK: C he's walking to baby shop [PP] and buy some chips.

LN/LE: C look at that one [PP].

.....

C XX (cause he's run) cause he's run off [PP].

References

King, G. and Fletcher, P. (1993) Grammatical problems in school-age children with specific language impairment. *Clinical Linguistics and Phonetics* 7 (4), 339–52.

Miller, J and Chapman R. (1981) The relation between age and mean length of utterance in morphemes. *Journal of Speech and Hearing Research* 24, 154–61.

Radford, A. (1988) *Transformational Grammar*. Cambridge: Cambridge University Press.

9 Acquisition of Negative Polarity Items

CHARLOTTE KOSTER AND SJOUKJE VAN DER WAL

Negative polarity items (NPIs), such as *any* and *ever*, are `lexical items or idiomatic expressions with a distribution in sentences which is not completely predictable from their syntactic properties' (Ladusaw, 1979). NPIs cannot appear in just any configuration; they must be licensed. In most cases, the licenser is some sort of lexical negative element (i.e. *no, not, nobody, never, none, nowhere*, etc.), as in examples (1) and (2), in which the NPIs are licensed in the negative sentences, but not in the corresponding affirmative ones:

(1) **any**   I don't want any soup.

                         *I want any soup.

(2) **ever**   None of us has ever been to Paris.

                         *All of us have ever been to Paris.

Obviously, the licensing of NPIs has something to do with negation, but overt negation is not the only possible licenser. There are other environments in which some NPIs are allowed, such as conditionals, questions, superlatives, or in the scope of certain adverbs, as is illustrated in the following examples with the NPI *ever*:

(3) **conditionals**   I shall kill you if you ever mention my visits here.

(4) **questions**   Have you ever been to Paris?

(5) **superlatives**   This is one of the best novels ever written.

(6) **certain adverbs**   Only John has ever been to Paris.

The above examples of possible licensing environments raise the question as to what exactly counts as a licenser for NPIs. Do the licensers all have a certain characteristic in common? Some theoretical approaches have attempted to answer this question:

— Ladusaw (1979) has taken a formal semantic approach, in which the licensing of NPIs is directly related to the logical properties of certain expressions or structures.

— Linebarger (1980), in a syntactic/pragmatic approach, makes negation the central issue in the licensing of NPIs. In her account, NPIs can only occur in the immediate scope of negation (the `Immediate Scope Constraint').

— A syntactic approach, by Progovac (1994), defines polarity items within the framework of the Binding Theory. NPIs obey Principle A in that they must be bound by a licenser (negation) or an empty polarity operator.

The distribution of NPIs is extremely complex, not in the least because their behavior shows large variation, both language-internally and cross-linguistically. First of all, NPIs differ as to the set of environments in which they can appear (Zwarts, 1994). For instance, not all NPIs are allowed in questions, or in superlative constructions. Secondly, although NPIs are a universal phenomenon, languages may differ as to which lexical items are polarity sensitive. None of the above mentioned theories can as yet give a unified account that conclusively fits these complex facts.

NPIs in Language Acquisition

In our experimental work on the acquisition of NPIs, we have not, as yet, committed ourselves to one particular theoretical approach. The acquisition of NPIs is largely uncharted territory, and it is not clear which factors, be they semantic, syntactic or pragmatic in nature, enhance the acquisition of these items or make them problematic.

The question of first importance is: are children aware of the fact that NPIs have a limited distribution? If it can be assumed that the child does not get direct evidence about the way in which certain words and expressions can*not* be used, how will a child know that an NPI is restricted in its use?

Secondly, if it can be shown that the distribution of NPIs is constrained in the grammar of the child, the next question is: do children use NPIs in the same restricted way as adults, or do the child's restrictions on NPIs deviate in some way?

The study presented in this paper is concerned with the first question: are NPIs, as soon as they appear in child language, restricted in their use or not?

An Early NPI: *hoeven*

In this study, the focus is on the verb *hoeven*, since it is the first NPI to appear in the language of Dutch children. *Hoeven* has no exact equivalent in English, but the verb *have to* or the modal auxiliary *need* comes close in meaning (cf. (7) and (8)):

(7)   Je mag het wel doen, maar het *hoeft* niet.

       You may do it, but you don't *have to*.

(8)   Hij *hoeft* niet te gaan.

       He *need* not go.

Hoeven is clearly an NPI in Dutch; it is only allowed in a restricted set of environments, such as negative sentences, comparatives, or in the scope of certain adverbs. It cannot be used in a straightforward affirmative sense; in that case, the verb *moeten* (*must*) should be used. *Moeten* is in meaning almost equivalent to *hoeven*, but differs from it in that it is not polarity sensitive; there are no particular restrictions on its use.

How is *hoeven* used in the spontaneous speech of Dutch children? We have carried out an investigation in a corpus of 18 children[1] from 0;11 to 3;10, which yielded many occurrences of *hoeven* directly followed by the negation *niet* (*not*). Some examples are given in (9)–(11) below:

(9)   1;08.06   Ik hoef niet.

                  I need not.

                  'I don't want to.'

(10)   2;00.12   Dirje hoeve niet handje   Sinteklaas.

                  Dirje need not little-hand Sinteklaas.

                  'Dirje doesn't want to shake hands with St. Nicholas.'

(11)   3;01.17   Hoeft niet gordijnen dicht.

                  Need not curtains closed.

                  'The curtains don't have to be closed.'

These examples are very representative of the way in which *hoeven* is used until the age of four. Although several other lexical items that can normally function as licensers were already present in the speech of these children (like *nothing, nobody, never,* etc.), they were not used in combination with *hoeven*. So, these examples show indeed a very restricted use of *hoeven*. It seems as if *hoef(t) niet* is used as a frozen expression, a general phrase for refusal or rejection of something.

Sometimes, however, *hoeven* is used improperly, in non-licensing environments. The following recorded child utterances are all ungrammatical in adult Dutch:

(12) 3;01.12   *xxx koffie. ik hoef .. dat koffie. xxx kouwe .. koffie.

                    xxx coffee. I need .. that coffee. xxx cold .. coffee.

                    'xxx coffee. I want that coffee. xxx cold coffee.'

(13) 2;04.11   *Hoef pappa fiets! (shaking her head)

                    Need daddy bicycle!

                    'I want to sit on daddy's bicycle!' (head shaking = *not*)

(14) 2;11.20   *Ik hoef van jou zachte 'n.

                    I need from you soft one.

                    'I want a soft one from you.'

(15) 3 years   *Ik hoef déze. (walking out of the garage with shovel in his hand)

                    I need this one.

                    'I'll take this one.'

From the contexts in which they were uttered, one can infer that these, for adults ungrammatical, utterances sometimes are meant to be negative, and sometimes affirmative. In example (12) for instance, it is probable that the child does *not* want cold coffee, although there is no negation present in the sentence. In example (13), where *hoeven* is used without a licenser, but is accompanied by head shaking, the father actually reported that the meaning was clearly negative. In (14), the sentence most probably has an affirmative meaning. In example (15), as in (13), more of the context is known and the meaning of this sentence with unlicensed *hoeven* was definitely affirmative.

In examples like (14) and (15), it is intriguing to see that, although *hoeven* is not properly licensed, the licenser may be hidden somewhere in the context, or in previous discourse. We will come back to this later.

A Child's Knowledge of *hoeven*

The spontaneous speech data seem to give the impression that children do not properly understand the negative polarity aspects of *hoeven*. Based on these observations, several questions can be formulated about how young children interpret this verb.

First, is it so that *hoeven* is known to young children only as a frozen expression with *niet* (*not*), as suggested by examples (9)–(11)? Or do children have a more complete understanding of *hoeven*, as an NPI, and of its various licensers? To investigate this possibility, it is necessary to look at a wider range of grammatically acceptable licensers, beyond the *niet* (*not*) that occurs in the spontaneous speech data.

A second hypothesis is whether *hoeven* alone possibly functions as a negative verb, with negation implicit in the verb — such that *hoeven* means *need-not*, as in (12) and (13). In this case, experimental investigation must focus upon what interpretation children give to *hoeven* when no licenser is present in the sentence.

Yet another hypothesis is that young children just see *hoeven* as a regular modal verb, like *moeten*. If *hoeven* is not an NPI for these children, then it could be used either negatively, as in (9)–(11), or affirmatively, as in (14) and (15). So again, it is necessary to find out what interpretations children give these sentences and, also, whether they see them as grammatically acceptable or not.

Of course, a fourth hypothesis is also possible: that children really do understand *hoeven* as an NPI, with specific restrictions on its usage.

An Experimental Study of *hoeven*

These possible explanations were tested via experimentation. So far, 11 three-year-olds have participated in this study. The children were tested with the Elicited Reproduction In Context task (ERIC) and an Acting Out task (AO). The task went as follows. One experimenter told the child a story, for example: *Bert's school is not so far away. Sometimes Bert goes there by bike, and sometimes he walks. What shall he do today? Bert says...* Then the other experimenter said the (in this case, for adults ungrammatical) test sentence for Bert: **I need to bike to school today*. The child was told to join in the storytelling by repeating what Bert had said (the ERIC response) and then to act out (the AO response) what Bert should do, with the help of toys or pictures.

The ERIC task is based partially on the standard Elicited Imitation task for children (Lust *et al.*, 1986). The motivation behind this task is that children will reproduce sentences in a way that fits their grammar. What the children are asked to do in this experiment is different from Elicited Imitation in that (1) the sentences are put in context; (2) ungrammatical, at least for adults, as well as grammatical sentences are presented; (3) via Acting Out, the child's interpretation of the sentence can be observed. Also, the child's attention is drawn away from a straightforward imitation instruction.

Via the ERIC response, the child's determination of acceptability is measured by his tendency to replicate or change the original sentence. Any changes made during reproduction give valuable information about where the grammatical shoe pinches, so to speak.

The ERIC task in combination with the AO task has specific advantages for the present investigation. For example, the story-test sentence pair illustrated above, with the ungrammatical test sentence **I need to bike to school today*, was paired with two pictures: Bert bicycling and Bert walking. The child, in the ERIC response, could a) give an exact repetition of the ungrammatical sentence; b) make the sentence grammatical by exchanging *hoeven* for a non-restricted, regular verb; or c) make it grammatical by inserting an acceptable licenser. The AO response shows the child's affirmative or negative interpretation. This, in combination with the ERIC response, gives the information necessary to interpret the child's understanding of *hoeven*.

There were 15 story-test sentence pairs and 15 story-filler pairs. Of the test sentences, there were 3 each of the grammatical types *hoeven-only*, as in (16a), *hoeven-no*, as in (16b), and *hoeven-not*, as in (16c).[2] There were also 6 ungrammatical sentences, in the sense that *hoeven* appeared without any proper licenser, the *licenser-absent* sentences, as in (16d) below:

(16a)   Ik hoef van jou alleen de gele te hebben.

          I need from you only the yellow to have.

          'I want only the yellow one from you.'

(16b)   Van de juf hoef ik geen rood potlood te slijpen.

          Of the teacher need I no red pencil to sharpen.

          'The teacher says I don't have to sharpen the red pencil.'

(16c)   Ik hoef de gele viltstift niet.

          I need the yellow marker not.

          'I don't want the yellow marker.'

(16d)   *Ik hoef vandaag naar school te fietsen.

          I need today to school to bicycle.

          'I want to bicycle to school today.'

Results

The graphs below represent three different result categories of the experimental data.[3] Figure 9.1 shows how often, in percentages, a child repeats the test sentence with either the verb *hoeven* preserved (repeated) in the ERIC response, or *hoeven* replaced by a different verb, like *moeten* (*must*), which is not an NPI.

What is immediately obvious is that, in repeating a *licenser-absent* sentence (16d), the children had a strong tendency to replace *hoeven* with a different verb, 40% of the time, which turns these sentences into grammatical utterances. In the sentences with *only*, *no* and *not*, (16a), (16b), and (16c), children more often than not repeated these sentences with the preservation of *hoeven*: 50%, 67%, and 80% of the time.

Figure 9.2 shows whether the child repeats, changes, or drops the

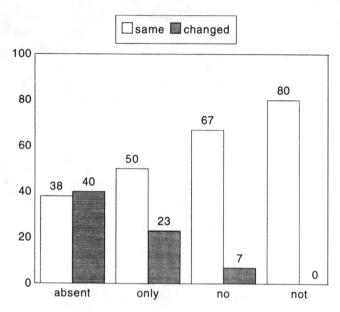

Figure 9.1 ERIC responses: verb same or changed.

licenser during the ERIC response. For example, in sentences with *not*, children repeated *not* 80% of the time, and used another, but still negatively interpretable licenser, such as *no* or *never*, 3% of the time, for a total of 83% negative licensers. They never replaced *not* with a different, affirmatively interpretable licenser like *only*, and dropped the licenser only 7% of the time. In the *licenser-absent* sentences, children repeated the sentences without a licenser 78% of the time, inserted an affirmatively interpretable licenser (like *only*) or 'pseudo licenser' (like *too* or *enough*; we will come back to this in the discussion) 8% of the time, for a total of 86% affirmative ERIC responses. They inserted a negative licenser (like *no* or *not*) 8% of the time.[4]

What we see in Figure 9.2 is, in comparison to spontaneous speech, when children of this age say only *hoef-not*, in their ERIC responses they are quite good at reproducing all these NPI licensers. It is the case, however, that they are most comfortable with *not*.

Figure 9.3 shows the children's Acting Out responses. The sentences with no licenser present (the *licenser-absent* sentences), and the *only* sentences were both acted out in the affirmative: 85% and 83% of the time. The *no* and *not* sentences should have both resulted in a negative interpretation. This was indeed the case 80% of the time for *not*, but the results for the *no* sentences were a bit of a surprise. A more complete investigation of this matter must wait for future research.

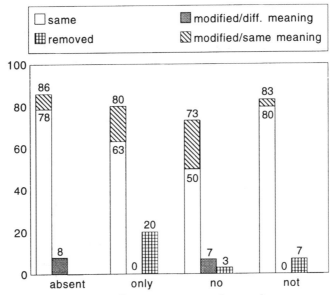

Figure 9.2 ERIC responses: licenser same or changed.

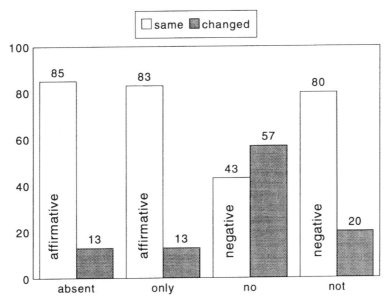

Figure 9.3 AO responses.

Discussion

What has this experimental investigation shown about children's knowledge of *hoeven* as an NPI? First, is there support for the hypothesis that *hoeven* is only known as a fixed negative expression, together with *not*? No: Figure 9.1 shows that, while the verb *hoeven* fares the best in the *not* sentences, there is no sharp contrast between the reproduction of *hoeven* in the *not*, *no* and *only* sentences. Also, in Figure 9.2, both the licensers *only* and *no* are preserved in the ERIC responses for the majority of these sentences.

Second, is *hoeven* without a licenser understood as an implicit negative verb? No: Figure 9.3 shows that *licenser-absent* sentences are acted out affirmatively 85% of the time.

Third, is *hoeven* considered to be just a regular modal verb? Again, no: as Figure 9.1 has shown, children are just not comfortable with an NPI verb in *licenser-absent* sentences. They replace *hoeven* in these sentences with other, grammatical verbs.

What about the fourth hypothesis about *hoeven*? The experimental evidence points in this direction. Three-year-olds do already seem to have knowledge of *hoeven* as a special verb, an NPI, with restricted use.

But then why do children sometimes use *hoeven* in ways that are deviant to adult language? A second look at the spontaneous speech examples, together with some of the more `original' ERIC reproductions, can give some insight into why children sometimes produce ungrammatical (according to adults) *hoeven* sentences.

Firstly, children seem to use negation or contrast in the context or in previous discourse as a licenser for *hoeven*, as in examples (14) and (15), presented earlier, in which there is a contrast between hard and soft pieces of clay (14), and a shovel or a broom (15). In both cases, the child chose between two alternatives, one of which was *not* needed, but the other was. Some other examples can illustrate this contextual or previous discourse licensing of *hoeven* (cf. (17)–(19)):

(17) 3 years   *Deke oef je niet, kete oef je wel.

                  Blanket need you not, kettle need you yes.

                  'You don't need the blanket, you do need the kettle.'

(18) 3;06.03   *Ik hoef nog niet naar bed, ik hoef nog eten.

                  I need yet not to bed, I need yet eat.

                  'I don't have to go to bed yet, I want to eat first.'

(19) 5;07.30   *Je hoeft hem toch wel te hebben?

                  You need him yet well to have?

                  'You do want to have it, don't you?'

In (17), the negation is in the first part of the sentence. Again, there is a situation in which there is a choice between alternatives; one is *not* needed, but the other is. In (18), the contrast is between going to bed, which is *not* needed, and having to eat first, which is needed. And lastly, in example (19), there may be a negation hidden in the context. It is as if the child has reason to believe that the person he is talking to does *not* need the object of the sentence. Now that the first experimental results have given some impression of the three-year-olds' basic understanding of the restrictions on *hoeven*, it should be possible to design an experiment that includes a more systematic investigation of the effects of contrast and discourse bias.

Secondly, in spontaneous speech data and the ERIC responses, children also use words that have the 'flavour' of licensers, but that are not real licensers: *wel*, *nog*, and *toch*, as for example in (17), (18), and (19), respectively. It is not yet clear why these words seem acceptable to children as licensers.

Thirdly, in the few cases where we found *hoeven* with the licenser *absent* in utterances with a negative meaning, we tend to think that these examples are performance errors: there are often pauses or unclear speech noted in the spontaneous examples at the spot where the licenser should have been. Also, in our experimental study, we found very little negative Acting Out of the *licenser-absent* sentences.

Conclusion

The main acquisitional problem for the child seems to be discriminating what the exact licensing environments are for the verb *hoeven*. In spontaneous speech data, most violations of polarity restrictions may be due to the intermediate grammar of the child, in which the concept of NPI-licenser has not yet been worked out in proper detail. Exactly what it is that the child does not control in relation to his understanding of *hoeven* and its licensing environments is, as yet, unclear. But what is now clear is that children do know is that *hoeven* is a special verb that must, in some way, be licensed.

Notes

1. Several corpora were used, some of which are available in the CHILDES database (MacWhinney, 1990): G. Bol and F. Kuiken, *the GRAMAT corpus*; L. Elbers and F. Wijnen, *the Utrecht corpus*; S. Gillis, *the Antwerp corpus*; F. Wijnen, *the Peter Files*; F. Wijnen and H. Veenhof-Haan, *the Wijnen corpus*.
2. The stories preceding the *hoeven-only* sentences (16a) introduced a weak story bias against the test sentence, and the stories preceding the *hoeven-no* sentences (16b) introduced a medium counterbias. The *hoeven-not* sentences (16c) were paired with preceding stories that introduced a strong bias against the test sentence interpretation. The possible effects of this bias are discussed in Van der Wal and Koster (1994).
3. The percentages do not necessarily add up to 100% per sentence here, because, for the sake of clarity, not all the scoring categories are presented in the Figures

(for example, minimal utterances, irrelevant acting out responses, etc.).
4. It should be pointed out that these Figures are not independent from each other. For example, look at Figures 9.1 and 9.2. First: contrary to what the 7% removed licenser for *not* sentences in Figure 9.2 might suggest, it is **not** the case that children turn grammatical *hoeven-not* sentences into ungrammatical *licenser-absent* sentences. These 7% removed *not*'s are in the missing 20% from Figure 9.1 — usually minimal utterances without any verb or licenser. Another example are the 20% removed *only*'s in Figure 9.2. Again, children did not turn grammatical *hoeven-only* sentences into ungrammatical *licenser-absent* sentences. Children dropped the *only*'s in the sentences where they also changed the verb — the 23% in Figure 9.1. Third, contrary to what the 78% repeated sentences without a licenser in Figure 9.2 seem to suggest, the children did show sensitivity to the restrictions on *hoeven* by changing the verb in these ungrammatical sentences — the 40% in Figure 9.1.

References

Ladusaw, W.A. (1979) Polarity sensitivity as inherent scope relations. PhD thesis, University of Texas, Austin.

Linebarger, M.C. (1980) The grammar of negative polarity. PhD thesis, Massachusetts Institute of Technology.

Lust, B., Chien, Y.-C., and Flynn, S. (1986) What children know: Methods for the study of first language acquisition. In B. Lust (ed.) *Studies in the Acquisition of Anaphora*. Vol.2. Dordrecht: Reidel.

MacWhinney, B. (1990) *The CHILDES Project: Computational Tools for Analyzing Talk.* Pittsburgh: Carnegie Mellon University.

Progovac, L. (1994) *Negative and Positive Polarity. A Binding Approach*. Cambridge: Cambridge University Press.

Van der Wal, S. and Koster, Ch. (1994) The negative side of polarity: Children's notion of licensing. In H. de Swart, H. de Hoop and A. de Boer (eds) *Language and Cognition* 4. Groningen: RUG.

Zwarts, F. (1994) Three types of polarity. Unpublished manuscript, RUG.

10 What Factors Predict a Child's Language in a Bilingual Environment?

JEAN LYON

Introduction

There are many questions still to be answered in the field of language acquisition, but the field of *bilingual* language acquisition is even less well explored. For a start, 'bilingual' is a word which most people use freely, but which is very difficult to define. It is connected with the speaking of two languages and it is used to describe societies and individuals. One of the major issues here is whether knowledge of two languages, or use of two languages is more important for this definition. Saussure (1916) first described langue (the knowledge of language) and parole (the use of language) as interacting but separate aspects of language development. Knowing is not the same as doing.

Grosjean (1982) focused on language usage. He is critical of attempts to follow Bloomfield's ideas and give bilinguals a 'balance' score (Bloomfield, 1933). These attempts have usually taken place in a controlled situation, ignoring the social context of language. The performance of any one individual varies according to who they are talking to, which language is the medium, and where they are at the time (Fishman, 1965). Immigrants may use only their first language at home and only the language of the community at work. Their bilingualism is different from that of children whose parents use two languages at home. These children may have grown up using one language only with their mother and a second only with their father. For them the parent is the language context.

Parents such as those described above were some of the first to study their own children's bilingual language acquisition. One of the earliest reports came from Ronjat describing the progress of his son, Louis, who by age 30 months, could use and understand simple French and German (Ronjat, 1913). Later, Leopold published four books of data about his daughter's bilingual language acquisition, this time English and German (Leopold, 1949a; 1949b; 1954 {originally published 1939}). With both children, their mother's language was stronger, at least initially. Later examples include Saunders, 1982; Taeschner, 1983; Fantini, 1985. Almost no work has been done using a normal population of children acquiring two languages informally. Parents with a special interest in language are a special group. Although they do usually attend to the language context of child language use, they do not represent ordinary bilingual language acquisition.

A few researchers have tried to suggest types of bilingual family (for example, Schmidt-Mackey, 1971; Romaine, 1989). These too have been based on those few cases which have been reported rather than on any survey of kinds of bilingual family which might exist in a given community. There probably exists a range of bilingual and monolingual families as there exists a range of bilingual and monolingual individuals.

McLaughlin's suggestion (1978) that, if children use two languages before age three they can be said to have acquired language bilingually, has been adopted generally. This is useful but the term can cover a wide range of youngsters, some of whom may have no more than a few words in a second language. Dodson (1983) calls this group 'developing bilinguals'. Some work has been done with schoolage children, but little with preschool children. It is suggested that the investigation needs to start in the early years in order to identify why some children become bilingual and some do not.

Method

Initially, parents on Anglesey in North Wales were sent a Language Background Questionnaire, QI, shortly after the birth of a baby. This asked about the language each parent used for a variety of activities and with a variety of people both currently and in the past. It had been decided that Language Use was a better measure than Language Knowledge.

From these replies, it was possible to divide families into five Language Background groups as follows (see Lyon, 1991 for details);

WW   Both parents use Welsh almost always.

WM   Mother uses Welsh primarily and Father does not.

MM   Both parents use a mixture of Welsh and English.

WF   Father uses Welsh primarily and Mother does not.

EE   Both parents use English almost always.

These families were sent a second questionnaire, QII, when their children were three years old, and their replies showed that they remained largely in their original grouping.

At QII, parents answered questions on 18 aspects of language use for each child, nine in Welsh and nine in English. From these replies (N = 124) it was possible to assign children to three groups, those using entirely or mostly Welsh (the monolingual Welsh group), those using entirely or mostly English (the monolingual English group), and those using both languages roughly equally (the Bilingual group).

Results

Current language background of monolingual and bilingual three-year-old children

It was expected that children who were reported to use only one language at age three, would have monolingual backgrounds and that those who were bilingual would come from one of the three mixed language backgrounds, WM, MM or WF. As can be seen in Table 10.1, most children fitted this pattern.

Table 10.1 Current language background of monolingual and bilingual three-year-old children

Background Children	WW	WM	MM	WF	EE	% of Total (N=124)
Welsh Mono.	88%	3%	3%	6%	0%	27%
Bilingual	12%	36%	38%	10%	5%	34%
English Mono.	0%	0%	27%	0%	73%	39%

That is, of the children who were monolingual English speakers at 3 years old, 73% were from EE backgrounds and 27% were from MM backgrounds. Those children comprised 39% of the total sample.

73% of the children who were monolingual English users at three lived in EE families, 88% of monolingual Welsh users lived in WW families and 84% of Bilingual children lived in families where both languages were used. In other words, the majority (81%) of all children lived with parents whose language use reflected their children's language development. But more than a quarter of the monolingual English children lived in MM families where both parents could use both languages, and more bilingual children came from WW families than from EE families (12% compared with 5%).

Early language background by child membership of language use group subsequently

The data were then examined prospectively. Table 10.2 looks at what happened to the children from the original language backgrounds.

Table 10.2 Early language background by child membership of language use group subsequently

Children Background	Welsh-Monolingual	Bilingual	English-Monolingual
WW	73%	27%	0%
WM	15%	75%	10%
MM	0%	30%	70%
WF	16%	58%	26%
EE	2%	10%	88%

This table emphasises the subsequent language use of children by early background. Thus, 73% of the children whose original language background was classified as WW (Welsh speaking), were found to be monolingual Welsh speakers at age three. The remaining 27% were bilingual.

As expected, most children from EE families became monolingual English speakers (88%) and none of the children from WW families did so. Those children became monolingual Welsh speakers mostly (73%), or else bilingual (27%). The MM group produced mostly English speakers (70%) and bilinguals (30%), and more than half of the children from WF and WM backgrounds became bilingual. A WF background seems more likely to produce monolingual English speakers than a WM background, but numbers are small in both of these groups, making generalisation hazardous.

Language background at birth seems to have some predictive value regarding the subsequent language development of the child. A WW background tends to lead to Welsh speaking, an EE background to English speaking and the other three groups tend to produce either bilingual children or English speakers.

Features of language use in the homes of monolingual and bilingual three-year-old children

Parents were asked about their language usage for a number of activities in QII. At this time, their children were three years old. They were also asked about the language/s heard and understood by the children, and the results are shown in Table 10.3.

It is hardly surprising that the majority of monolingual children heard their first language mostly and were said to understand it. Similarly, it is hardly surprising that the majority of bilingual children hear and understand both languages at home. However, most of their parents use Welsh as a first language.

Table 10.3 Features of language use in the homes of monolingual and bilingual three-year-old children

		Welsh	*Bilingual*	*English*
Language	Mostly W.	95%	53%	0%
Parents Use	Both	2%	32%	30%
	Mostly E.	2%	16%	70%
Language	Mostly W.	98%	60%	1%
Child Hears	Both	2%	39%	41%
	Mostly E.	0%	2%	58%
Language	Mostly W.	93%	26%	1%
Child	Both	5%	70%	5%
Understand	Mostly E.	2%	4%	94%

Percentages of children classed as Welsh speaking, Bilingual or English speaking according to parental language use, language heard and language understood at home.

Interesting as well is that many (41% of) English monolingual children hear Welsh spoken, whereas very few Welsh monolingual children either hear or understand English.

Multiple regression analyses

Variables from QI and from QII were entered into a series of multiple regression analyses. As can be seen in Table 10.4, the independent variables were taken from the first questionnaire, completed shortly after the children were born, and the dependent variables from the second questionnaire which was completed around the time of the children's third birthday.

It had been expected that the language background of the family (or Couple Language) would be the best predictor of a child's later language, but this was not so. In the summary of the results (Table 10.5) neither couple language nor any of the maternal wishes or beliefs had much predictive value. Maternal language accounted for by far the most variance in each of the regression analyses performed, although paternal language did contribute to each of these analyses independently.

Table 10.4 Variables used in multiple regression analyses

INDEPENDENT VARIABLES

(from Questionnaire I at child's birth)

1.   MATERNAL LANGUAGE USE

2.   PATERNAL LANGUAGE USE

3.   COUPLE LANGUAGE (Language Background)

4.   MATERNAL WISHES (for child Welsh learning)

5.   MATERNAL IMPORTANCE (importance assigned to Welsh)

6.   MATERNAL OPINION (about the future of Welsh)

7.   MATERNAL MARRY (hopes regarding child marriage)

DEPENDENT VARIABLES

(from Questionnaire II when child was 3 years old)

1.   DEVELOPMENT of WELSH

2.   DEVELOPMENT of ENGLISH

3.   DEVELOPMENT of BILINGUALISM

4.   LANGUAGE CHILD USES

5.   LANGUAGE CHILD UNDERSTANDS

Discussion

At age three, most children who were monolingual lived in families who were also monolingual or virtually monolingual. Bilingual children mostly lived in families where both parents used a mixture of languages, or where one parent was primarily a Welsh speaker and the other primarily an English speaker. These results are what one would expect.

However, more than a quarter of the monolingual English speaking children came from mixed language (MM) backgrounds, and more bilingual children came from Welsh speaking homes than from English speaking homes. It would seem that children are more likely to learn English than Welsh when both languages are in the home, and more likely to learn English than Welsh as a second language if they come from a monolingual background.

These conclusions are supported by an examination of original backgrounds. Again, monolingual backgrounds tend to produce monolingual children and families where two languages are used tend to

Table 10.5 Summary of multiple regression analyses

(Dep.Vars) (Indep.Vars)	Develop Welsh	Develop English	Develop Biling.	Lang. Child Uses	Lang. Child Understds
Maternal Language	52%	41%	58%	64%	57%
Paternal Language	5%	12%	10%	10%	14%
Couple Language	–	7%	3%	2%	–
Maternal Wishes	1%	–	–	–	–
Maternal Importance	–	–	–	–	2%
Maternal Opinion	1%	3%	–	–	1%
Maternal Marry	–	1%	1%	–	1%

MATERNAL LANGUAGE when the child was born accounted for most of the variance (from 41% to 64%)

PATERNAL LANGUAGE also made a small but independent contribution.

produce bilingual children (Table 10.2). However, Welsh monolingual backgrounds are more likely to produce bilingual children than are monolingual English families, and mixed language families are more likely to produce English speaking than Welsh speaking children.

The languages heard and understood by children are largely consistent with their language group. However, more bilinguals hear mostly Welsh and more English speaking children hear both languages than the Welsh speaking group. It would seem that this last group is somehow able to avoid aural contact with English more easily than the other groups avoid Welsh. As both languages are rife, it is possible that parents of Welsh speaking children have actively attempted to delay their children's contact with the English language. Or else that they are less aware of the pervasive nature of English.

The multiple regression analyses show clearly the influence of maternal language use on the language use of three year old children. This was not expected. As the design of the research indicates, the language background was originally thought to be the most powerful influence on child language. Fathers have an independent influence on their child's language, but the language used by the mother at the start of the child's life best predicts his or her future language use, at least at age three.

Summary

Parents from families in North Wales reported the language development of their children in both Welsh and English at age three years. Measures were available on 18 aspects of language, nine in Welsh and nine in English, making it possible to assign children to three groups, mostly monolingual Welsh, Bilingual and mostly monolingual English.

Results were mostly as expected, with monolingual children living in monolingual families and bilingual children living in families where both languages are used. There was, however, some evidence that the English language is more often learned by children from monolingual Welsh and two language families than Welsh is learned by children from these or monolingual English families.

Comparisons were made between parental opinions, parental language use, and the Language Background of the family at the time when the child was born, and that child's subsequent language use at three years old. As expected, this showed that families where both parents were primarily Welsh-speaking (WW) tended to produce monolingual Welsh speaking children, and those with primarily English speaking parents (EE) tended to produce monolingual English speaking children.

Using data from the time of the children's births, multiple regression analyses were performed to discover which factors best predict a child's language at three years old. Although fathers have some influence on their children's language, by far the greatest predictor of future language use is the mother's language when the child is born.

References

Bloomfield, L. (1933) *Language*. London: Allen and Unwin.
Dodson, C.J. (1983) Living with two languages. *Journal of Multilingual and Multicultural Development* 4, 401–14.
Fantini, A.(1985) *Language Acquisition of a Bilingual Child: A Socio-linguistic Perspective*. Clevedon: Multilingual Matters.
Fishman, J.A. (1965) Who speaks what language to whom and when? *La Linguistique* 67–68.
Grosjean, F. (1982) *Life with Two Languages*. Cambridge, MA:Harvard University Press.
Leopold, W. (1949a) *Speech Development of a Bilingual Child; A Linguist's Record. Vol.III; Grammar and General Problems in the First Two Years*. Evanston, IL: NW University Press.
— (1949b) *Speech Development of a Bilingual Child; A Linguist's Record. Vol.IV; Diary from Age Two*. Evanston, IL: NW University Press.

— (1954 {1939}) *Speech Development of a Bilingual Child; A Linguist's Record. Vol.I; Vocabulary Growth in the First Two Years*. Evanston, IL: NW University Press.

Lyon, J. (1991) Patterns of parental language use in Wales. *Journal of Multilingual and Multicultural Development*. 12 (3) 165–83.

McLaughlin, B. (1978) *Second–Language Acquisition in Childhood*. Hillsdale, NJ: Lawrence Erlbaum.

Romaine, S. (1989) *Bilingualism*. Blackwell: Oxford.

Ronjat, J. (1913) *Le Development de Langage observe chez un Enfant Bilingue*. Paris: Champion.

Saunders, G. (1982), *Bilingual Children; Guidance for Families*. Clevedon: Multilingual Matters.

Saussure, F. (1916) *Cours de Linguistique Generale*. Paris: Payot.

Schmidt-Mackey, I. (1971) Bilingual strategies of bilingual families. In W. Mackey and T. Anderson (eds) *Bilingualism in Early Childhood*. Rowley, MA: Newbury House .

Taeschner, T. (1983) *The Sun is Feminine; A Study on Language Acquisition in Bilingual Children*. Berlin: Springer-Verlag.

11 The Nature of Children's Initial Clauses[1]

ANDREW RADFORD

This chapter presents a structure-building account of the acquisition of clause structure, focusing mainly on children acquiring Ll English. I argue that the earliest clause structures produced by English-acquiring children are VPs, and that a VP analysis can provide a straightforward account of numerous aspects of the morphosyntax of early child clauses. For example, I suggest that null subjects are null constants which can be discourse-identified by virtue of occupying a root (VP-) specifier position; and similarly that early verbs are intrinsically nonfinite, and can be assigned discourse-determined temporal reference by virtue of being root constituents. I also argue that scopal (negative and interrogative) constituents occupy VP-adjunct position, and hence precede clause subjects. I go on to posit that there is evidence of a VP stage in the acquisition of other languages (e.g. Mauritian Creole). I suggest that children develop from an initial VP stage to an ultimate CP stage via an intermediate IP stage, and argue that UG principles determine how children come to project VP into IP and CP. In the case of interrogative structures, I argue that principles relating to scope and structural economy determine that wh-phrases will be moved into the minimal structural position in which they have scope over the rest of their clause. Thus, children will initially adjoin wh-phrases to VP (in nonergative clauses); at the later IP stage, they will adjoin them to IP; and once they start to use complement clause questions (and IP adjunction is barred for complement questions by the no-adjunction-to-arguments constraint), they will move wh-phrases into their ultimate landing-site in the specifier position within CP (though IP adjunct position will remain available as an alternative wh-landing site in root clauses for a while.)

1. Introduction

This paper is concerned with the nature of the earliest clause (i.e. subject+predicate) structures produced by one-year-old children: for ease of reference, I will refer to these as CICs (viz. Children's Initial Clauses). At the stage in question (which they typically go through somewhere between one-and-a-half and two years of age), children acquiring L1 English produce verbal clauses headed by a nonfinite verb,[2] as illustrated by the examples in (1–3) below (the name and age in years and months of the child producing each utterance is given in parentheses):

(1) Baby talking (Hayley 1;8)
  Doggy barking (Bethan 1;9)
  Daddy coming (Helen 1;9)
  Wayne sitting on gate (Daniel 1;9)
  Mummy doing dinner (Daniel 1;10)

(2) Daddy gone (Paula 1;6)
  Wayne taken bubble (Daniel 1;9)
  Jem drawn with Daddy pen (Jem 1;11)
  Mummy thrown it (Jem 1;11)
  Bunny broken foot (Claire 2;0, from Hill, 1983)

(3) Paula play with ball (Paula 1;6)
  Bethan want one (Bethan 1;8)
  Machine make noise (Kathryn 1;9, from Bloom, 1970)
  Hayley draw boat (Hayley 1;8)
  Baby eat cookies (Allison 1;10, from Bloom, 1973)

One analysis of CICs like (1–3) (suggested in Radford, 1986, 1990; Lebeaux, 1987, 1988; Guilfoyle & Noonan, 1988; Kazman, 1988; Vainikka, 1993) posits that they are *Small Clause* (SC) constituents which are simple projections of a head nonfinite lexical V constituent, so that children's clauses at this stage have a structure along the lines indicated in (4) below:

(4)

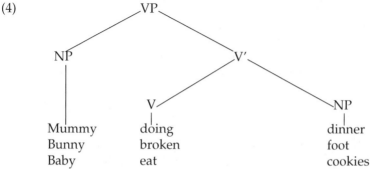

All theta-marking takes place under sisterhood, in that the complement is θ-marked by the head V, and the subject is θ-marked by its sister V-bar constituent.[3]

Under the SC analysis, *all* children's clauses at stage I are VPs which are direct projections of argument structure. It follows from this assumption that early child clauses have no functional architecture, and thus lack IP and CP projections. Evidence for the non-projection of IP comes from the fact that children make no use of infinitival *to* or auxiliaries at this stage; for example, in contexts where adults require an IP headed by infinitival *to* (with an overt or null subject) children use a simple VP, as illustrated by the following examples taken from a longitudinal study of a boy called Daniel:

(5) Want [have money] (1;7)   Want [Teddy drink] (1;7)
      Want [open door] (1;8)   Want [Dolly talk] (1;9)
      Want [go out] (1;10)   Want [lady get chocolate] (1;11)

Likewise, corresponding to adult negative clauses containing the finite auxiliary *do*, children typically produce auxiliariless negative structures such as those in (6) below (from the Nina files on the CHILDES data base):

(6) No my play my puppet (2;0.2)   No lamb have it (2;0.3)
      No dog stay in the room (2;1.2)   No Leila have a turn (2;1.3)

Evidence for the non-projection of a CP constituent in CICs comes from the fact that children's earliest complement clauses such as those in (7) below lack complementisers:

(7) Want [Baby talking] (Hayley 1;8)   Want [Mummy come] (Jem 1;9)
      Want [this go up] (Angharad 1;10) Want [lady open it] (Daniel 1;10)

and from the fact that they omit complementisers on sentence-repetition tasks (cf. Phinney, 1981). Further evidence comes from the fact that they do not produce structures containing inverted auxiliaries; for example, the earliest interrogative clauses produced by Jane (a child studied longitudinally by Hill, 1983) at age 24–25 months included structures such as the following:

(8) Chair go? Kitty go? Car go? That go? Jane go home? Mummy gone?

The adult counterpart of *Jane go home?* would be *Did Jane go home?*, with the preposed auxiliary *did* occupying the head C position of CP. The fact that children's clauses do not contain complementisers or inverted auxiliaries at this stage is consistent with the hypothesis they are producing Small Clause (VP) structures which lack a CP projection.

If we assume that a clause is a projection of a lexical verb (as argued by Jackendoff, 1974, 1977; Williams, 1975; Bresnan, 1976 and Abney, 1987) then VP structures are 'clauses' in the same way as IP and CP structures are: in the terminology of Radford, 1993, V is the *ultimate head* of the clause; in the terminology of Grimshaw, 1991, IP and CP are *extended projections* of V. There are some parallels between children's nonfinite VP structures and what Akmajian (1984) terms *Mad Magazine* (MM) sentences, i.e. sentences such as that italicised below:

(9) - You've been cheating on me, admit it.
     - What? *Me cheat on you*? Never!

The parallel with MM sentences extends to the fact that the latter appear to be simple VP projections headed by a nonfinite verb with an oblique subject, and do not allow IP constituents like *to* (cf. 'What? *Me to cheat on you*? Never!'). Moreover, like child SCs, adult MM sentences allow null subjects with variable reference (cf. 'What? Deprive *myself/yourself/himself* of creature comforts? Never!').

Since it first appeared, the Small Clause Hypothesis (SCH) has been attacked by a number of linguists on three main grounds, namely (i) lack of *descriptive adequacy* (in that SCH fails to provide an adequate account of the morphosyntax of particular phenomena in early child grammars, e.g. interrogatives, negatives, null arguments, case, etc.); (ii) lack of *universality* (in that SCH is incompatible with known facts about the acquisition of languages with a more complex morphosyntax than English), and (iii) lack of *explanatory adequacy* (in that SCH presupposes an essential discontinuity between adult and child grammars, and fails to explain why early child clauses should be 'smaller' than adult clauses, or how children's 'small clause' VPs develop into adult 'full clause' CPs. In place of the SCH, a variety of alternative *functional* analyses have been proposed in which all or some functional projections are 'in place' from the very earliest clauses which children produce. In each of the sections below, I answer specific criticisms which have been levelled at SCH, and compare SCH with alternative *functional* analyses of CICs. For the most part, the data I consider in this paper will relate to the L1 acquisition of English; however, section 7 discusses the applicability of the SCH to other child languages.

2. Null Subjects

A well-known characteristic of early grammars is that between a third and a half of CICs have null subjects (as noted e.g. by Hyams 1986 and much subsequent work). Typical null subject CICs are illustrated in (10) below:

(10) Want that. Want Lisa. Want baby talking (Hayley 1;8)
      Want one. Gone out. Got it. Lost it. Coming to rubbish (Bethan 1;8)
      Want crayons. Want biscuit. Want mummy come. Pee in potty (Jem 1;9)
      Find Mommy. Taste cereal. Close . . . door. Go house. Sit lap (Kendall 1;10, from Bowerman, 1973)
      Make arms. Make pineapple. Making one (Kathryn 1;10, from Bloom, 1970)
      Want tiger. Get tiger. Shoot Tina (Domenico 2;0)

Opponents of SCH have argued that it is essential to posit the existence of a CP and/or IP projection is order to provide a principled account of how null subjects are licensed and identified in CICs. For the sake of brevity, I shall confine myself to just one such 'functional' account of early null subjects, namely that in Hyams 1994 30–38 (for an earlier functional account, see Pierce, 1989 and Déprez & Pierce, 1993, 1994).

Hyams makes the following three assumptions:

(11) (i)   *pro* is (universally) licensed in A positions in initial grammars
     (ii)   spec-CP is an A-position if occupied by a subject (since it will be construed with the agreement features carried by INFL)
     (iii)   null root specifiers can be discourse-identified.

Given her analysis, a sentence such as 'Want teddy' (meaning 'I want my teddy') would have a structure along the lines of (12) below:[4]

(12) $[_{CP} \, pro_i \, \text{COMP} \, [_{IP} \, t_i \, \text{INFL}_i \, [_{VP} \, t_i \, [_V \, \text{want}] \, \text{teddy}]]]$

The null subject *pro* is raised into spec-CP (root specifier position), and is coindexed with INFL (by virtue of the fact that its trace stands in a spec-head agreement relation with INFL). Hyams (1994: 33) maintains that 'The null element in spec-CP is associated with and identified by a discourse topic through a process of *topic chaining*'; discourse identification is made possible here by virtue of the fact that the null subject is in spec-CP (root specifier position — cf. (11)(iii) above).

There are a number of aspects of Hyams' spec-CP analysis of null subjects which are potentially problematic. For example, the assumption that INFL carries abstract subject-agreement features raises the question of why these don't surface on the verb morphology at this stage (i.e. why children don't make productive use of the 3SG affix +s). Moreover, the assumption that a null subject raises *vacuously* from spec-IP to spec-CP is in conflict with constraints against vacuous movement (such as that suggested in Chomsky, 1973) and with the principle of *economy of derivation* argued for in Chomsky, 1988. It also poses learnability problems and flies in the face of Chomsky's (1986: 50) hypothesis that 'The language learner assumes that there is syntactic movement only where there is overt evidence for it' — indeed all the more so as Hyams assumes *vacuous* movement of a *vacuous* (i.e. null) constituent.

No less troublesome is the problem raised by Hyams herself (1994, fn. 13, p. 48) of how to deal with children's null-subject wh-questions such as:

(13) Where going?

If the null subject in (13) is in spec-CP, where is the wh-phrase *where* positioned, given the standard assumption that wh-phrases are positioned in spec-CP? Hyams answer is to suggest that 'Sentences such as (13), which are apparently rare, are derived via adjunction of the wh-phrase to CP'. Thus, the price which Hyams has to pay for attaining a unitary (spec-CP) analysis of null subjects is a fragmentary analysis of wh-movement under which wh-phrases move to spec-CP in sentences with overt subjects, but adjoin to CP in sentences with null subjects. Given that adult English does not license wh-adjunction to CP,[5] this makes for obvious *discontinuity* between child and adult grammars.

Still, if null-subject wh-questions are indeed 'rare', then we might argue that structures such as (13) are peripheral in child grammars — perhaps the result of a performance (e.g. spellout failure) error. But this raises the question of precisely how *rare* such structures are. Null-subject wh-questions are widely reported in the acquisition literature. For example, Klima and Bellugi (1966: 200) report *What doing?* as a typical stage I question: Plunkett (1992: 58) reports that one of the earliest wh-questions produced by her son was *Where go?*; and Vainikka (1993) provides the following examples of null subject wh-questions produced by Adam, and Eve:

(14) Where put? (Eve 1;9)   Where go? (Adam 2;3)
      What say? (Adam 2;4)   Where find plier? (Adam 2;4)
      Where go drop it? (Adam 2;4)

Moreover, if we look at the corpus of utterances produced by Jane at age 24 months (in Hill, 1983), we find Jane producing null-subject utterances such as *What doing?* and *Where go?* In actual fact, 39% [11/28] of Jane's questions containing overt wh-words have null subjects. Thus, the claim that subjectless wh-questions are 'rare' seems a doubtful one and yet such questions are problematic for Hyams' analysis.

But how does the Small Clause analysis account for early null subjects? Under the SC analysis, a sentence such as *Want Teddy* would have the structure (15) below (where *ns* is a syntactically projected empty category representing the null subject):

(15) [$_{VP}$ *ns* [$_V$ want] Teddy]

If, following (11)(i), we assume that null subjects are licensed in A positions, then the null subject in (15) is licensed by virtue of the fact that it occurs in spec-VP. Moreover, if we assume (following (ll)(iii)) that a null constituent can be discourse identified in a root specifier position, then since *ns* occupies a root specifier position in (15), it can be discourse identified.[6]

Interestingly, the analysis in (15) is also compatible with the account of the identification of early null subjects in Rizzi (1992, 1993, 1994). Rizzi argues that early null subjects (in the case of children acquiring non-null-subject languages) represent a type of null definite description which he calls a null constant *nc*. He argues that *nc* must be Ā bound by a non-quantificational operator, but that binding requirements hold only if they are satisfiable in principle. It then follows that *nc* will be exempt from the binding requirement only where it occupies a position where it cannot be so bound, i.e. only in a root specifier position.

But what of null subject wh-questions such as those in (14)? Anticipating the discussion in section 6 below, let us suppose that wh-phrases in CICs are adjoined to VP, so giving rise to structures such as the following (where *e* is an empty category bound by *where*):

(16) $[_{VP}$ Where $[_{VP}$ *ns* $[_V$ go] *e*]]

Since the null subject *ns* occupies root specifier position, it is both licensed (by virtue of being in an A position) and discourse identified (by virtue of being in a root specifier position). Thus, null-subject declaratives and interrogatives alike can be readily accommodated within the SC analysis.

3. Tense Binding

A further objection which might be made to the analysis of early child clauses as root nonfinite VPs relates to the fact that nonfinite clauses typically cannot function as root clauses in adult grammars, arguably because (according to Zagona, 1988) nonfinite verbs must be *tense-bound* (i.e. bound by a c-commanding tensed constituent).[7] We might then argue that a functional analysis of CICs such as (17)(b) below is to be preferred to a lexical VP analysis such as (17)(a):

(17) (a) $[_{VP}$ Wayne $[_V$ sitting] on gate]
     (b)   . . . INFL$_i$ $[_{VP}$ Wayne $[_V$ sitting$_i$] on gate]

(. . . here indicates the possible presence of additional functional architecture above INFL, though since it plays no part in the discussion here, it is omitted). The reason for preferring the functional analysis (17)(b) would be that given such an analysis, the nonfinite verb *sitting* would be bound by an INFL constituent (which we might assume to carry abstract tense properties), whereas under the VP analysis (17)(a), the nonfinite V *sitting* is unbound. Thus (it might be claimed) only (17)(b) is consistent with principles of UG.

There are a number of problems with this argument, however. If INFL carries tense properties, how come these are not realised either on an item in INFL, or on the head V of VP (via I-lowering, V-raising, or V/I agreement?). Conversely, if (following Wexler, 1994) we assume that early INFL has no tense properties at all, how can the nonfinite verb be tense-bound by a tenseless INFL? More importantly still, we might question whether a root nonfinite VP does indeed need to be tense-bound. An alternative view would be to suppose (following Chomsky and Rizzi) that binding requirements only hold *where they are satisfiable in principle*. Under the SCH, we can then argue that root nonfinite verbs do not need to be tense-bound at this stage precisely because they cannot be so bound in principle (given that children at this point in their development project no tensed constituents which could bind untensed verbs). It would then follow that the temporal reference of root nonfinite verbs would be discourse-identified — just as the reference of null root subjects in CICs is discourse identified.[8]

4. Case

Pierce (1989) argues that we need to posit an abstract INFL constituent in CICs in order to account for how the subject receives case. She proposes that early child clauses contain an abstract INFL constituent which assigns nominative case (via government) to the subject in spec-VP, in the manner schematized in (18) below:

(18) ... INFL [$_{VP}$ *Teddy* [$_V$ want] sweetie]
     |------------↑

She posits that 'INFL is "present" and can assign nominative case structurally to the VP-internal subject in early grammar' (pp. 58–59).

There are both theoretical and empirical problems posed by this analysis, however. The major theoretical problem is that nominative case assignment is canonically associated with a *finite* INFL: given that the child's verbs are nonfinite at this stage, and that a nonfinite INFL (e.g. infinitival *to*) is not a case assigner, how can INFL assign nominative case? The solution which Pierce suggests is that INFL carries no specific *tense* properties at this stage, and that 'INFL which is not explicitly specified for a + or – tense feature assigns nominative case by default' (Pierce, 1989: 59). However, if INFL carries neither tense nor agreement at this stage, what function does it serve (given that the classical view of INFL is as a constituent which carries tense and agreement)? The answer is that it serves no other function than that of providing a mechanism by which the subjects of clauses can be assigned (default) nominative case: moreover, the mechanism invoked (case assignment via government by INFL) is not one which is operative in adult English, so that the analysis involves developmental discontinuity. Thus, the postulation of an abstract INFL is a purely *ad hoc* construct with no independent motivation, and no explanatory value.[9]

As noted above, the 'abstract INFL' analysis also faces empirical problems. A core assumption of the analysis is that a subject in spec-VP is assigned *nominative* case by INFL. An immediate potential problem for this claim comes from the numerous studies which show that subjects of CICs frequently surface with oblique (i.e. objective/genitive) case as noted by Radford, 1986: 20–22, Kazman, 1988: 11–12, Aldridge, 1989: 82–5 (and as is clear from examples of objective subjects cited in many earlier works such as Gruber, 1967; Menyuk, 1969; L. Bloom, 1970; Huxley, 1970; Brown, 1973; etc.). Typical examples (from Radford, 1986: 21 and Vainikka 1993: 9) are given below:

(19) Me talk (Stephen 1;7)   Me do it (Bethan 1;8)
     Me have biscuit (Angharad 1;10)   My close it. My get my car (Nina
     1;11) My need her. My make red table (Nina 2;0)

Replying to this objection, Nina Hyams (1992b: 373) remarks that 'Such errors are rare'. But is this so?

In a careful statistical study of the acquisition of case-marking, Anne Vainikka (1993) argues to the contrary. For example, she notes that only 11% of the lSG subjects used by Nina from age 1;11 to 2;1 were nominative *I*, the remainder being oblique subjects (predominantly genitive *my*, but also two instances of *me*). In Radford (1986), I reported that early pronominal subjects used by the children in my corpus typically carried objective case. The fact that subjects surface with objective or genitive case (alongside nominative case)[10] poses a potential problem for the INFL analysis. If we adopt Pierce's analysis and suppose that INFL uniformly assigns syntactic nominative case to the subject in spec-VP, it seems that we have little choice but to follow Halle and Marantz (1993: 171, fn. 9) and 'allow morphosyntactic features to be changed at MS' [Morphological Structure]; we might then suppose that syntactic nominative case is variously realised as morphological nominative, objective, or genitive case. Such a solution clearly has minimal explanatory value, and poses obvious learnability problems (e.g. How does the child delearn the objective and genitive realisations of syntactic nominative case?).

Consider now how we might account for the case-marking of subjects under SCH.[11] There are three possibilities which we might envisage — that the subject is assigned *structural case*, *inherent case*, or *default case*. Vainikka (1993: 6) proposes a structural account of genitive subjects, arguing that children extend the process by which N licenses a genitive specifier to other lexical heads, so that V too licenses a genitive specifier: cf. her remark that 'Genitive can be assigned not only by N but also by V . . . Genitive case is assigned structurally by these heads to an NP in the specifier position of the case assigner': cf also Lebeaux, 1987: 36 who adopts a similar analysis. Radford (1992a: 240) outlines a structural account of the case marking of objective subjects, suggesting that SC subjects are assigned objective case by virtue of standing in a spec-head relation with an untensed (nonfinite) verb. If (following Roeper & de Villiers, 1992) we assume that young children at this stage have not yet acquired (cross-clausal) Exceptional Case Marking (ECM), then it may be that children infer from ECM structures such as 'Let [*me* have one] that nonfinite verbs license objective subjects.[12] A residue of this 'nonfinite objective subjects' rule would then persist into the adult grammar in gerund constructions such as '*Him* turning up late was really irritating', and in 'Mad Magazine' sentences such as 'What? *Me cheat on you*? Never!'

An alternative possibility is to suppose that the subjects of CICs carry *inherent* case — i.e. case assigned to constituents as a function of the thematic role which they fulfil. This position is reflected in interesting work by Nancy Budwig (1984, 1985, 1989). She notes that the youngest children she studied alternate between the use of nominative, objective and genitive subjects like *I/me/my*, and observes (1984: 5) that: 'The uses of *my* link up with utterances in which the child acts as a prototypical agent bringing about a change (for instance: *My blow the candles out* and *My do it*), while those containing *I* (for example, *I like peas* and *I no want those*) deviate from the agentive perspective.' She observes that 'The use of *I* is found most often in utterances expressing the child's experiential states and intentions'. She also notes (p. 6) that in utterances with *me* subjects, 'The child refers to self as a subject *affected* by action.' A natural interpretation of her observations is that that the relevant children assign inherent case to subjects, with prototypical AGENTS being assigned genitive case, prototypical EXPERIENCERS nominative case, and prototypical PATIENTS objective case.

A variant of the inherent case analysis would be to assume that case reflects *argumenthood*, so that (e.g.) internal arguments (in VP complement position) receive objective case, and external arguments (in VP specifier position) receive genitive case (or perhaps nominative case for some children). For the children reported in Radford 1986 who assign objective case to subjects and complements alike, we might suppose that any thematic argument of a verb is assigned objective case.

Under either variant of the *inherent case* analysis, case is directly correlated with thematic/argument structure. Such a correlation would provide an account of why the subjects of ergative predicates frequently surface in postverbal position in CICs such as the following (from Pierce, 1989: 78–79):

(20) (Here) come Eve (Eve 1;7)   Come Fraser (Eve 1;8)
     All gone grape juice (Eve 1;7)   Going (re)corder (Naomi 1;10)
     Go Foster in town (April 2;9)   Come Cromer? (Adam 2;5)
     Broken car (Adam 2;4)

The postverbal position of ergative 'subjects' can be accounted straightforwardly (as noted by Pierce, 1989: 81) if we assume that children directly project lexical entries onto morphosyntactic structures (and if we further assume that ergative 'subjects' are internal arguments). A second phenomenon which we can thereby account for is the observation made by Hyams (1986: 63) that CICs are characterised by 'a notable lack of . . . expletive pronouns'. Such pronouns would be absent precisely because they have no thematic role to play, and hence cannot be assigned case and so are unlicensed. We might conjecture that expletives trigger subsequent acquisition of structural case marking of subjects, and at this point inherent case-marking of subjects is catapulted out of the grammar (to use the metaphor developed in Randall, 1992).

Amy Pierce (1989: 62) briefly discusses the idea that arguments are assigned inherent case in early grammars, but dismisses it on the grounds that 'Case assignment which overlaps with theta role assignment is vacuous as a licensing condition'. But against this, we might object that any grammar in which case-marking directly reflects theta-marking is surely optimal. For example, a direct mapping from theta structure into case structure would satisfy the *Isomorphism Principle* posited by Hyams (1986: 162) which requires that grammars maximise the structural isomorphism between different levels of representation. What the *inherent case* analysis predicts is that children should have few problems learning the case assigned to complements (because this is thematically determined), but would have potential problems learning the case assigned to subjects (since this is syntactically determined). And indeed, this prediction seems to be borne out: thus, not only do children have problems with assigning case to finite subjects, but in addition, Roeper & de Villiers (1992) present experimental evidence that case-marking for the subjects of exceptional clauses is late-acquired. Independent support for this claim comes from the observation made by Chiat (1981: 86) and Kazman (1988: 11) that children frequently produce exceptional infinitive clauses with nominative subjects such as those bracketed below:

(21) Let [he go in your bed] (Sally 2;4)
       Let [she go on your swing] (Sally 2;4)
       See [he walk] (Peter, no age specified)

and from the observation by Nishigauchi and Roeper (1987: 119, fn. 19) that some young children produce complement clause structures such as:

(22) Help [*my* eat it]   See [*my* ride it]   See [*my* do it backwards]

One interpretation of data such as (21) and (22) is that for the children concerned, there is a direct mapping from thematic/argument structure onto morphosyntactic structure: the complement clause subject is assigned case as a function either of its thematic role (e.g. genitive because it is an AGENT), or of its argument status (e.g. nominative because it is an external argument).

A final possibility would be to assume that SC subjects receive *default* case: more particularly, we might suppose that by virtue of being arguments they must be made visible through case, and that when they occupy a position which is not inherently case-marked, they receive default (objective) case (cf. the proposal to the effect made by Roeper & de Villiers, 1991: 8–10 and 1992: 220). It might be argued that a *default case* account involves no developmental discontinuity in that objective case also serves a default function in adult grammars: e.g. in contexts where a nominal receives neither nominative case, nor genitive case, nor null case, objective case is assigned by default (so accounting for the objective case carried by pronominal sentence fragments (cf. 'Who did it? — *Me*') and by the subjects of 'Mad Magazine' sentences (cf. What? *Me* cheat at cards? Never!). It goes without saying that the *default* analysis is applicable only to objective subjects (not to nominative or genitive subjects, for which an alternative account has to be developed).

Of course, it might be objected that an account which sees the oblique case marking of subjects as determined by their thematic/argument structure status can easily be 'grafted' onto an IP account. If this is done, it follows that INFL plays no role in assigning case to spec-VP. But if INFL carries no tense properties, no agreement properties and no case properties (i.e. none of the criterial properties of INFL), what motivation is there for assuming that it is present at all?

5. Negation

The earliest type of (non-anaphoric) negative structures produced by young children are typically presubject negatives, as illustrated by the examples in (23) below (from Pierce, 1989: 93–4; Déprez & Pierce, 1993: 34, and Déprez & Pierce, 1994: 61):

(23) Not Fraser read it (Eve 1;9)   No I see truck (Adam 2;3)
      No the sun shining (Adam 2;4)   No Butch is gonna walk (Peter, 2;2)
      No my play my puppet, play my toys (Nina 2;0.2)
      No Mommy doing. David turn (Nina 2;0.2)
      No lamb have it. No lamb have it (Nina 2;0.3)
      No dog stay in the room. Don't dog stay in the room (Nina 2;1.2)
      No Leila have a turn (Nina 2;1.3)

Déprez and Pierce (1994: 61) report that of the earliest negative sentences produced by Eve at ages 18–21 months, Peter at 23–25 months and Nina at age 23–25 months, 96% (71/74) contained sentence-initial negatives.

Nina Hyams (1992b:379) proposes a functional analysis of presubject negatives under which *no/not* are analysed as an INFL constituents (i.e. as negative auxiliaries), so that a child sentence such as *No Fraser drink all tea* would have the structure (24) below:

(24) ... [$_I$ No] [$_{VP}$ Fraser [$_V$ drink] all tea]

However, there are a number of reasons for being sceptical about such an analysis. For one thing, *no/not* don't have the selectional properties of typical auxiliaries, in that they take a range of different (infinitive/ progressive/perfective) complement types, as we see from:

(25) Not *do* it (Stefan 1;8)
      Not *doing* it (Bethan 1;8)
      Not *done* it (Hayley 1;8)

By contrast, it is a criterial property of auxiliaries (and indeed of all functional heads, according to Abney, 1987) that they select a specific type of complement (e.g. in adult English, modals select an infinitive complement, progressive *be* selects an +*ing* complement, perfective *have* selects an +*n* complement, etc.). Moreover, if *no/not* are auxiliaries, we would expect them to behave like typical auxiliaries in allowing elliptical complements — and yet we don't find children using structures such as

(26) *Daddy not/no*

as elliptical clauses (e.g. to mean 'Daddy can't find it'). Furthermore, we would also expect that if *no/not* are auxiliaries, they will undergo inversion — and yet child negative questions such as:

(27) *No(t) he coming?* ['Isn't he coming?']

are unattested. What's more, if *no/not* were (finite) auxiliaries, we would expect them to license only nominative subjects — but this would leave us with no obvious way of accounting negative sentences with oblique subjects such as the example 'No *my* play my puppet' cited in (23) above. The auxiliary analysis would also lead us to expect that (at least some) children would attach the 3SG present affix +*s* or the past tense affix +*d* to *no/not* — and yet child sentences such as those in (28) below:

(28) Daddy *noes/noed/nots/notted* help me

are unattested. Moreover, the auxiliary analysis would entail the postulation of an obvious discontinuity between child and adult grammars, in that the child has (somehow) to delearn her miscategorisation of negatives as auxiliaries. In short, the INFL analysis of *no/not* provides us with more questions than answers.

Pierce (1989), and Déprez & Pierce (1993, 1994) offer an alternative functional account of early child negatives in which they posit that children generate nonanaphoric *no/not* negatives in spec-NEGP, so that an utterance such as *No Mommy doing* has the S-structure (29) below (cf. Déprez & Pierce, 1993: 36 and 1994: 62):[13]

(29) . . . INFL [$_{NEGP}$ No NEG [$_{VP}$ Mommy [$_V$ doing]]]

However, such a structure is far from unproblematic. They assume that the subject (*Mommy*) is assigned structural nominative case under government by INFL. However, this poses two problems. One is that case assignment via head-government is subject to a strict adjacency condition, whereby any constituent intervening between the *case-assigner* and the *case-assignee* blocks case assignment: e.g.

(30) I sincerely *believe* **him** to be unsuitable for the post
     *I *believe* sincerely **him** to be unsuitable for the post

(31) *Will* **she** definitely be there?
     Will* definitely **she be there?

Why, then, does NEGP not create a barrier to case marking of the subject by INFL in structures like (29)? Why doesn't the subject raise from spec-VP to spec-IP to receive case via spec-head agreement, and hence appear in front of the negative? Given that INFL does not assign case to spec-VP under head government in adult English, the analysis carries an inherent assumption of discontinuity between adult and child grammars.

Having shown that functional accounts of early negation are unsatisfactory, let me now turn to consider how we might account for early negative sentences under the Small Clause analysis. Hyams, 1992b: 378 claims that 'There does not seem to be any easy way of accommodating external negation into the small clause analysis.' I shall argue here that on the contrary, the SC analysis permits us to arrive at a straightforward analysis under which the syntax of early negatives is determined by UG principles. Let us suppose (following Kazman, 1988: 17; Guilfoyle & Noonan, 1988: 37; Lebeaux, 1988: 39 and Radford, 1990: 154) that negatives are generated as VP-adjuncts, so that a sentence such as *No Fraser sharpen it* will have the structure (32) below:

(32) $[_{VP}$ No $[_{VP}$ Fraser $[_V$ sharpen] it]]

One of the UG principles which 'guides' the child to analyse negatives as clausal adjuncts is the *Isomorphism Principle* posited by Hyams (1986: 162) which specifies that grammars maximise the structural isomorphism between different levels of representation. Hyams herself notes that this principle will account for the position of negation: if we assume that the child identifies negatives as operators which must have scope over (and hence c-command) the entire clause at LF, then it follows that the Isomorphism Principle will determine that negatives occupy preclausal position at S-structure as well, in order to maximise the isomorphism between LF and S-Structure.

However, a second UG principle which plays a central role in determining the locus of negation is the following:

(33) *Minimal Projection Principle*[14]
    S-structures are the minimal well-formed projections of the lexical items they contain

As noted by Grimshaw (1993a: 5), it follows from a principle such as (33) that 'A clause is only as big as it needs to be. It is an IP unless it has to be a CP (a VP unless it has to be an IP).' One effect of this principle is to *minimise extended projections* (Recall that IP and CP are extended projections of V: cf. Grimshaw, 1991). This would mean (e.g.) that in negating a simple (VP) projection such as *Fraser sharpen it,* the child will not develop an extended projection in which *no(t)* is generated as the specifier of an abstract functional projection FP, as in (34) below:

(34) $[_{FP}$ No $[_F]$ $[_{VP}$ Fraser $[_V$ sharpen] it]]

The reason is that the FP structure (34) will violate the *Minimal Projection*

Principle (33), since the VP structure (32) is simpler by virtue of being a *simple projection* (i.e. (32) is a single headed projection of V), whereas the alternative functional structure (34) is a more complex *extended projection* (i.e. it is a double-headed projection of F and V). In terms of the Minimal Projection Principle (which leads children to prefer single-headed structures to multiple headed structures), we can *explain* the observation made by Solan and Roeper (1978), Roeper 1992 and Hoekstra and Jordens (1994) that children's initial strategy for incorporating new material into a clause is to adjoin it to the overall clause.

A final point to note in connection with the VP-adjunct analysis of early child negative sentences is that we maximise continuity with adult grammars, given the arguments by Zanuttini (1989) that *not* is a VP-adjunct in adult English.

6. Wh-Questions

Children's CICs typically contain a very limited range of wh-questions. Leaving aside potentially formulaic copula questions such as *What(s) dat?*,[15] the earliest wh-questions produced by young children are typically wh-complement questions (i.e. questions in which the wh-word is the complement of a verb) of the form *What NP do(ing)?* or *Where NP go(ing)?*. For example, Klima & Bellugi, (1966) report sentences such as *What cowboy doing?* and *Where horse go?* as the earliest wh-question types produced by Adam, Eve and Sarah. Bowerman's (1973) transcripts of Kendall's speech at 23 months includes the questions *'Where doggie go?'* and *'Where pillow go?* The corpus included in Hill (1983: 119–141) contains the following examples of verbal questions with overt wh-complements and overt subjects produced by Jane at age 2;0.[16]

(35) Where girl go? Where pencil go? Where cow go? (x2) Where Daddy go? Where bathtub go? What kitty doing? What the dog doing? What squirrel doing? What lizard doing?

Once wh-structures become more productive, we find a wider range of wh-complement questions, as illustrated by the following set of examples produced by Adam at age 2;4 (from Vainikka 1993: 34):

(36) Who me tickle? What say? What dat tell her? Where dat come from? Where find plier? Where go drop it? (Adam 2;4)

As noted earlier in relation to the examples in (8) above, a well-known characteristic of early wh-questions is that children at this stage do not make use of the presubject auxiliary found in adult questions — and the obvious question to ask is 'Why?'. The traditional answer is that auxiliaries in wh-questions in colloquial speech tend to be 'weak' monosegmental clitic forms, or even null forms: cf.

(37) Where'd he go? [= did]   Where's she live? [= does]
     What you doing?[= are]   Where you been? [= have]

Given the hypothesis (put forward by McNeill, 1966 and Gleitman & Wanner, 1982) that items which lack acoustic salience fail to be parsed by young children, it follows that the child's 'intake' (in the sense of White, 1982) for questions like (37) will be as in (38) below:

(38) Where he go? Where she live? What you doing? Where you been?

Thus, the absence of auxiliaries in early wh-questions is not difficult to account for. Moreover, if we assume that the child 'knows' that the wh-phrase is the complement of the verb, and that the canonical position of complements is postverbal, it follows that the child concludes that structures like (38) are CVS [= Complement+Verb+Subject] structures which involve movement of a wh-complement. But what is the landing site of the preposed wh-phrase?

Supporters of the *strong continuity hypothesis* argue that continuity considerations require us to assume that the landing-site for preposed wh-phrases is the same in Child English as in Adult English, i.e. that in each case the wh-phrase is moved into spec-CP. Given the 'strong continuity' assumption, a child question such as *What kitty doing?* will have the structure (39) below:

(39) $[_{CP}$ What$_i$ COMP $[_{IP}$ kitty$_j$ INFL $[_{VP}$ t$_j$ $[_V$ doing] v$_i$]]]

where t_i is the trace left behind by movement of the subject *kitty* from spec-VP to spec-IP, and where v_j is a variable bound by the moved wh-phrase *what$_i$*. Of course, advocates of 'strong continuity' might wish to go further and argue that (39) contains a null finite allomorph of progressive *be* which tense-binds the nonfinite verb *doing*, and that the auxiliary moves from INFL to COMP (as in adult English). On the continuity account, all the child would have to learn is how to spell out the auxiliary. In contrast — it is alleged — SCH can provide no convincing account of early wh-questions such as (35) and (36). Thus, Déprez & Pierce (1994: 75) maintain that 'The [SCH] view that the COMP projection is not present in the immature grammar leaves the well-known early acquisition of wh-movement unexplained'. They further comment (p. 77) that 'If spec-CP is the landing-site of wh-movement, as proposed by Chomsky 1986, then the early acquisition of overt wh-movement in child language suggests that COMP is available as a landing site — and at the earliest stage'.

However, the continuity account is far from unproblematic. One crucial learnability question which it leaves unanswered is how the child comes to identify spec-CP as the landing site for moved wh-phrases in English. It cannot be that principles of UG determine that spec-CP is the (universal) landing-site for moved wh-phrases, since there is strong evidence of parametric variation across languages with respect to wh-landing sites.

For example, Grimshaw (1993a) argues that in French root interrogatives, wh-phrases surface either in preverbal spec-CP position (as in (40)(a) below) or in presubject adj-IP (IP adjunct) position (cf. (40)(b)):

(40) (a)   *Qui* **a**-t-elle rencontré? 'Who **did** she meet?'
     (b)   *Qui* **elle** a rencontré? 'Who **she** did meet?'

Rudin (1988) and Kraskow (1994) similarly argue that both landing-sites are licensed in Slavic languages, so that we find structures with a wh-phrase moving to adj-IP — as in the following Polish example:

(41) Maria myśli, [$_{CP}$że [$_{IP}$ co [$_{IP}$ Janek kupił]]]
     Maria thinks that what Janek bought
     'What does Maria think that Janek bought?'

Moreover, Jimenez (1994) argues that wh-movement in Spanish (for non-discourse-linked wh-phrases) is to spec-IP. Thus, UG licenses at least three different landing-sites for preposed wh-phrases, namely spec-CP, spec-IP, and adj-IP. Indeed, our earlier discussion of subjectless wh-questions like (13) highlighted the fact that Hyams also needs to assume that wh-phrases can be adjoined to CP — which entails a fourth landing-site for wh-phrases. It would seem that the only generalisation which UG provides about the landing-site for preposed wh-phrases is that they are moved into a position where they have scope over (i.e. c-command) the overall interrogative clause. In this connection, it is interesting to note the suggestion by Penner (1992: 252) that the syntax of wh-phrases is determined by the following UG principle:

(42) *Scope Principle*
     Wh elements must be placed in a scope position either in the syntax
     or at LF

The problem which this poses for the continuity account is that a principle such as (42) will clearly not enable the child to pick out spec-CP as the landing-site for wh-movement, since (42) is compatible with a range of possible alternatives (e.g. movement to spec-IP, adj-IP, adj-CP, etc.). Learnability considerations require that we find some way of narrowing down the set of alternative landing sites which (42) makes available to the child. But what kind of principle will narrow down the hypothesis space for the child?

The answer provided by the Small Clause Hypothesis is that the relevant principle is the *Minimal Projection Principle* (33). This will interact with the *Scope Principle* (42) to determine that wh-phrases move into the minimal position in which they have scope over the overall clause. In the case of ergative structures like those in (20) above whose subjects remain in postverbal comp-VP (i.e. VP complement) position, spec-VP will be available as a wh-landing-site, so that we should expect to find (e.g.) *Where go train?* parallel to Eve's (1;7) *Here come Eve* cited in (20) above. For structures with an (overt or covert) subject in spec-VP, however, we expect wh-phrases to be adjoined to VP. Thus, the two types of wh-question we expect to find at this stage are of the schematic form indicated below:

(43) (a)   [$_{VP}$ Where [$_V$ go] train]
     (b)   [$_{VP}$ What$_i$ [$_{VP}$ kitty [$_V$ doing] e_i]]

In (43)(a), it is not clear whether *where* is directly projected into spec-VP, or moves into spec-VP from some underlying comp-VP (internal argument) position, thereby leaving behind an empty category in comp-VP; in (43)(b), e_i is an empty category bound by the wh-pronoun *what*.[17] The resulting structures (43) are *simple projections* of V, and hence will be favoured over any structure such as (39) which involves one or more abstract extended functional projections (IP and CP in the case of (39)). As in the case of negative particles, the S-structure location of wh-phrases is determined for the child by the interaction of UG principles relating to *scope* and *minimal projection*. By contrast (as we saw earlier), it is not obvious how the child determines the landing-site of preposed wh-phrases on Hyams' CP account.

7. Universality

Hyams (1994: 22) dismisses the SCH as a 'historical accident', arising out of the fact that proponents of SCH looked at the acquisition of English; she suggests that it is only the fact that English has minimal and nonuniform finite verb morphology and relatively rigid SVC [= Subject+Verb+Complement] word order which enables the SCH to account for CICs in English. However, she argues, if we look at the acquisition of (e.g. Romance or Germanic) languages with a richer verb morphology and verb syntax, 'We see that children acquire certain inflectional elements at a very early age, from the beginning of their multiword utterances. Moreover, they control syntactic operations such as verb raising and verb second (V2), which are dependent on the presence of functional heads' (Hyams, 1994). Hyams' claims would appear to be borne out by numerous empirical studies arguing that in the initial stages of the acquisition of other languages such as French (cf. Pierce, 1989), German (cf. Poeppel & Wexler, 1993) and Italian (cf. Guasti, 1992), children already differentiate finite from nonfinite verbs both in respect of their morphology and in respect of their syntax (in that finite verbs are positioned before negatives and nonfinite verbs after negatives, and clitics attach to the left of finite verbs but to the right of nonfinite verbs).

However, a word of caution needs to be sounded. The claim that there is a potential 'Small Clause' stage cannot be disconfirmed simply by taking an arbitrarily chosen corpus (of the speech of one or more children around two years of age), and demonstrating that the child/children in question has/have already acquired the morphosyntax of finite verbs.

After all, the fact that at time T_j (or during some period $T_j \ldots T_k$, $k > j$) a given child has acquired the morphosyntax of finite clauses does not preclude the possibility that an earlier time T_i ($i < j$) the child might not have done. The VP period is a *grammatical stage* characterised by a cluster of co-occurring grammatical properties (described in Radford, 1986), not a *chronological age*: while — as suggested in Radford, 1990 — most children seem to pass through this stage into the functional stage at around age 2;0 (± 20%), some do so earlier and others later (e.g. Vainikka, 1993 estimates that Eve passes out of the VP stage at 1;8, Nina at 2;1, Adam at 2;3, and Sarah at 2;4). Moreover, while some children go through an extended period (of 3 or more months) in which they produce only nonfinite clauses, for others this period may be much shorter — indeed vanishingly short if we espouse the possibility suggested by Roeper (1992: 340) that children may go through 'silent stages'. The fallacy of generalising from the observation that child X at age Y was not at stage Z to the conclusion that 'There is no stage Z' is self evident.

Instructive in this regard is Adone-Resch's (1990) study of the acquisition of Mauritian Creole (a language in which finiteness is marked by tense/aspect/modality auxiliaries). All the two-year-old children in her corpus show productive use of one or more auxiliaries (the earliest to be acquired being progressive *pe*, perfective *fin*, past *ti* and future *pu*). Supporters of FCH would no doubt invite us to conclude that here is additional evidence that children's earliest clauses contain functional categories. However, Adone-Reschs's data also show that the youngest child studied (Laura, age 21 months) produced no auxiliaries at all (She omitted them 33 times in obligatory contexts — cf. Adone-Resch, 1990: 98), leading Adone-Resch to the conclusion that 'She has not yet distinguished between finite and nonfinite verbs' (1990: 100), and that 'Children like Laura have not yet developed an IP' (1990: 110) . Typical utterances produced by Laura at age 1;9 (from Adone-Resch, 1990) are given below:

(44) Mami sufe 'Mummy blow'   Dada ale 'Daddy go'
    Vid delo '[I] pour water'   Mete '[I] put [it]'
    Peny atet '[I] comb head'   Aste to '[I will] buy sweet[s]'
    Pas ade sa '[I] Not look-at that' Pas one '[I] not know'

Thus, Laura turns out to be the crucial 'missing link' in the overall picture of development. The obvious conclusion to draw is that children like Laura have 'a syntax without functional projections' (Adone, 1993: 8).

Much the same can be said of Amy Pierce's (1989) study of the acquisition of French. She argues that the three children she studied show clear evidence of the acquisition of an IP constituent, in that they differentiate finite from nonfinite verbs both morphologically and syntactically (e.g. the negative *pas* 'not' is positioned before nonfinite verbs but after finite verbs). However, if we read her work carefully, we uncover the observation that in the very first recording of Nathalie at age 1;9;3 (designated by Pierce as N1/T1), Nathalie uses only nonfinite verb forms, not finite verbs. Thus, Pierce, (1989: 41) observes that 'Nathalie at N1 lacks tensed verbs', and concludes that there is an 'absence of inflected forms in the very early stages' (1989: 42), noting that 'In Nathalie at T1, then, we catch a glimpse of a stage in French acquisition before verb raising to tense sets in.' Thus, far from being 'freaks', children like Laura and Nathalie provide us with a crucial 'glimpse' (to use Pierce's own word) of an earlier Small Clause stage.

Hernández Pina's (1984) longitudinal study of her son Rafael acquiring L1 Spanish provides us with a further glimpse of the SC stage. She notes that the root clauses produced by Rafael from 18 to 24 months of age were often headed by nonfinite verb forms (infinitives, gerunds, and participles): cf.

(45) Nenes sentar 'Children sit+infinitive'
     Papa tuyando 'Daddy studying'(1;10)
     Roto caja 'Broken box' (1;10)

She also notes that during the same period Rafael produced a number of imperatives and 3SG present indicative forms such as:

(46) ¡Satata ab[r]e! '[Let] Fuensanta open [it]' (1;7)
     Mete dedo '[I] puts [my] finger [there]' (1;10)

Although it might be supposed that clauses like (46) are finite (and hence justify positing an IP projection), Pierce (1989) and Tsimpli (1992) argue that this is not so, pointing out that Rafael's verbs show no tense, agreement or mood contrasts at this stage (e.g. imperative and indicative verbs have the same form): both Pierce and Tsimpli argue that verbs occupy the head V position of VP, and that subjects are in spec-VP. If their claims are substantiated, it is plausible to suppose that Rafael's earliest sentences are Small Clause (VP) constituents.

Thus, one reply which might be given to Hyams' claim that SCH does not extend to languages other than English is that there are a number of published studies of the acquisition of languages other than English which point to a very different conclusion (evidence for a Small Clause stage has been reported for Swedish in Platzack (1990), for Greek in Tsimpli (1992), for French in Meisel (1992) and for German in Guilfoyle and Noonan (1988) and Meisel (1992)). However, let us suppose that at least some speakers of some languages don't pass through a visible Small Clause stage. Let us further suppose (for the sake of argument) that Echeverría (1978: 65) and Clark (1985: 713) are right in claiming that children's early clauses in Spanish show examples of CVS order alongside the dominant SVC order.[18] Let us also suppose (in the spirit of Koopman & Sportiche, 1991) that CVS structures involve movement of the verb to INFL and of the complement to spec-IP, so resulting in S-structures of the form (47) below:

(47) [$_{IP}$ Complement$_i$ [$_I$ Verb$_j$] [$_{VP}$ Subject [$_V$ t$_j$] t$_i$]]

If all these suppositions are well-founded, we would appear to have evidence for the early existence of at least some functional architecture above VP.

There are several questions which are raised by this kind of argumentation, however. The first question to ask is how the child comes to learn that V moves to INFL and that its complement moves to spec-IP. The only answer I can see that we can give to this question is to suppose that the child first learns to project thematic structure onto a canonical VP structure in which the subject is in spec-VP and the complement in comp-VP (i.e. in VP complement position); only after children have established the canonical position of subjects and complements within VP can they (in principle) come to 'realise' that structures in which the complement occupies noncanonical preverbal position and the verb occupies noncanonical presubject position are the result of movement into higher positions within a functional projection. In other words, *learnability* considerations lead us to conclude that the IP stage presupposes the existence of an earlier (perhaps 'silent') VP stage.

A second question which we need to ask about an analysis such as (47) is whether there is any evidence for positing the existence of a functional projection above VP. An alternative possibility (cf. Radford, 1994) would be to suppose that in order to accommodate the preposed verb and preposed complement, the child projects an empty 'shell' above VP — i.e. a projection whose head X carries no intrinsic categorial properties, so resulting in a structure such as (48) below:

(48) [$_{XP}$ Complement$_i$ [$_X$ Verb$_j$] [$_{VP}$ Subject [$_V$ t$_j$] t$_i$]]

If we assume that once X is filled by the preposed verb it inherits the categorial properties of the verb which it contains, then it follows that the resulting structure XP will have the derived categorial status of a VP. This means that (48) will be a 'stacked VP structure' at S-structure — not a functional IP structure. We might argue that movement of the complement into a superordinate specifier position is simply a focusing operation, and that movement of V to X is required in order to fill the head (i.e. to satisfy the constraint proposed by Gawlitzek-Maiwald *et al.* (1992) and Grimshaw (1993a, 1993b) that heads must obligatorily be filled. The moral of this story is that movement operations don't necessarily entail the postulation of functional projections.[19]

A final comment which needs to be made about the type of argumentation associated with structures such as (47) is the following. It follows from the *Minimal Projection Principle* (33) that children will project only the minimal structure needed to accommodate the lexical items in a given (child) sentence. As we have seen, for a language with a relatively impoverished verbal morphosyntax (e.g. English), a simple VP structure enables the child to project a wide range of clause structures (declaratives, negatives, interrogatives, etc.) at an early stage. However, for a language like Spanish with a much richer verbal morphosyntax, we might suppose that the child identifies at a very early stage that verbs carry a rich tense/mood/agreement morphology and can occupy noncanonical presubject position. We might therefore suppose that UG principles force the child learning such a language to project an IP constituent at the outset: this will be the case if UG principles require that verbs with a rich inflectional morphology raise to INFL. On such a scenario, only children acquiring languages with an impoverished verbal morphosyntax will be expected to show evidence of a visible Small Clause stage; for children acquiring languages with a rich verbal morphosyntax, we expect the Small Clause stage to be invisible. Thus, the conclusion we reach is exactly the opposite of that reached by Hyams, namely that the languages which teach us most about the earliest stages of acquisition are those in which verbs have a relatively impoverished morphosyntax, for example English.

8. Explanatory Adequacy

Given that the ultimate goal of any theory is explanatory adequacy, two crucial questions which the SCH has to answer are (i) *why* the earliest clausal structures developed by young children are lexical VPs, and (ii) *how* these early clauses subsequently develop into functional IP and CP structures.

A number of different answers have been given to the *Why VPs?* question. One is a *lexical learning* account, which holds that (in consequence of the *Minimal Projection Principle*) children project only those lexical items which they have acquired at any given stage of development, and that they acquire *contentives* before *functors*. It follows from these assumptions that their earliest clauses are projections of the four major categories of contentive — noun, verb, adjective and preposition. Of course, this account raises the question of why contentives are acquired before functors: typical answers given to this question are that functors are late acquired because of their lack of acoustic salience (Gleitman & Wanner, 1982: 17), or their greater cognitive/semantic complexity (Hyams, 1986: 82), or their greater grammatical complexity (Radford, 1990: 264–66), or the fact that they are subject to substantial parametric variation across languages (cf. the *functional parametrisation hypothesis* of Chomsky 1988).

A second type of explanation (cf. Radford, 1990: 266–68) is a *structural* (more specifically, teleological) one. We might argue that it is in the nature of the grammatical structure being acquired that some parts of the structure must be 'in place' before others can develop. For example if we adopt the view of Grimshaw (1991) that all clauses share a common VP 'core', and that IP and CP are *extended projections* of VP, then it follows that children cannot in principle develop IP or CP projections until they have developed VP.[20]

A third type of explanation which might be offered is a maturational one (cf. Cinque, 1988). That is, we might suppose that the principles which enable the child to project argument structures onto lexical syntactic structures (i.e. structures which are projections of lexical categories) come 'on line' at an early age (e.g. 1;6), whereas the principles which enable the child to form extended (functional) projections of lexical structures come on line somewhat later (e.g. 2;0).

Consider now the *How?* question — i.e. the problem of 'explaining how the functional categories are acquired if they are initially absent' (Hyams, 1994: 21). The problems posed for the SC analysis in this regard are very much parallel to those posed by any *functional* analysis which (like that of Pierce, 1989 and Déprez & Pierce, 1993, 1994) posits that subject, verbs and complements all remain within VP in CICs. Given lack of space, the account of development which I offer below is of necessity partial, and is limited to a discussion of the development of phrase structure (more specifically of the functional architecture in clauses).

Following Guilfoyle & Noonan (1988) and Vainikka (1993) let us suppose that the first stage after the VP stage is an IP stage (starting at around 2;0 and lasting for several months) during which VP has an extended projection into IP.[21] However, in keeping with the traditional assumption that when children first enter a 'new' stage they initially alternate between 'old' and 'new' structures, I shall assume that:

(49) When they first acquire a given type of functional extended projection, children only *optionally* project the relevant functional architecture

(Cf. the suggestion in Rizzi, 1993 that children between 2;0 and 2;6 *optionally* project functional categories). What this means is that when children first enter the IP stage, they alternate between projecting V into VP or IP, so that their clauses at this (second) stage are sometimes VPs, sometimes IPs.

The earliest type of INFL constituent developed by young children is typically an auxiliary of some kind: for example, Radford & Aldridge (1987) report on a group of children whose first INFL constituents were a subset of modal auxiliaries (and infinitival *to*). Pierce (1989: 85–9) suggests that copula/auxiliary *be* is the first INFL constituent to be acquired by Naomi.[22] Vainikka (1993) argues that the first INFL constituents produced by Nina are modals at age 2;1 (file 10) with past tense +*d* appearing (and being overgeneralised) at the same time (file 10), and the dummy auxiliary *do* appearing shortly afterwards (file 12). Nominative case is acquired at the same time as modals/tense (Nina produces only one *I* subject in file 9, but 56 in file 10), suggesting a direct correlation between the acquisition of tense and nominative case (cf. the claim by Watanabe 1993 that tensed verbs license nominative subjects). Vainikka notes (in relation to 1SG subjects) that modals are used only with *I* subjects, whereas nonauxiliary verbs are used with either nominative or oblique subjects: cf.

(50) *I* seed you (Nina 2;1, file 10)
    My ate outside (Nina 2;1, file 10)

She suggests that clauses with nominative subjects are IPs, and that clauses with oblique subjects are VPs. We might suppose that complement clauses at this stage can similarly be IP or VP constituents, so accounting for the fact that as the complement of verbs like *want* children use both infinitival IP complements headed by *to*, and *to*-less VP complements.

The IP/VP analysis makes interesting predictions about the syntax of wh-phrases. We might expect in the case of ergative predicates with postverbal 'subjects', spec-VP will be available to act as the locus for preposed wh-phrases (or for locatives like *here/there*), so giving rise to sentences like *Where go train?* or *Here come train*. In the case of predicates with preverbal subjects, we expect wh-phrases in VP structures to be adjoined to VP (as in stage I), with the subject in spec-VP carrying oblique case — and structures such as (51) below (from the CHILDES data-base) seem to represent this type of clause:

(51) *Who* me tickle? (Adam 2;4, file 4)
    What me write (Adam 2;10, file 16)
    Where me sleep? (Adam 2;11, file 17)
    Why me go? *Why* me going? (Adam 2;11, file 18)
    What my doing? (Eve 1;10, file 9)
    What my need? (Eve 2;0, file 13)
    Mommy, *where* my sit? (Sarah 3;0, file 40)
    How my bang my head? (Sarah 3;0, file 42)

But what of IP structures? Pierce (1989) and Déprez & Pierce (1993: 60 and 1994: 74) argue that the earliest auxiliaries used by young children do not trigger raising of the subject from spec-VP to spec-IP, so that the subject remains in spec-VP 'below' the auxiliary, even in declarative sentences such as:

(52) Is shoes off (Naomi 1;11.2) Is kitty sleep (Naomi 1;11.3)
    Is it hard (Naomi 1;11.3)   Is it broken (Naomi 1;11.3)

If the subject does not raise to spec-IP, it follows that spec-IP will be available as a landing-site for preposed wh-phrases, so resulting in WhAuxS (Wh-phrase+Auxiliary+Subject) structures such as (53) below in which the wh-phrase might be analysed as being in spec-IP and the (italicised) oblique subject in spec-VP.[23]

(53) Where is *him*? (Nina 2;5, file 29)
     How old are *me*? (Sarah 3;1, file 46)
     What's *them*? (Jonathan 2;4)
     Where's *me*? (Michelle 2;5, trying to find her picture in a photo album)

Indeed, the presumed spec-VP position of the subject may be the reason why the copula seems to agree with the preceding wh-phrase rather than the following subject in sentences such as (54) below, given that agreement is canonically a relation between INFL and spec-IP:[24]

(54) What colour is these? (Holly 2;0)
     What's the wheels doing? (Holly 2;0)
     Where's my pictures? (Nina 2;1, file 9)
     What's these? (Adam 2;2)
     What's these? What's those? (Jonathan 2;4)
     Where's my hankies (Katy 2;4)
     What's those? (Alistair 2;6)
     What's you doing? (Ellen 2;9)
     What's animals' names? (Kelly 3;0)
     Where is his feet? (Jonathan 3;3)
     Where is you? (Elspeth 3;3 = 'Where are you?')

We might further conjecture that early inverted yes-no questions such as (55) below:

(55) Is this doggie? (Naomi 1;10.19)   Is it raining? (Naomi 1;11.6)
     Is it gone? (Naomi 1;11.6)   Is it going to work? (Naomi 1;11.6)
     Can me have biscuit? (Angharad 1;10)

are IP structures in which spec-IP is occupied by a null yes-no question operator (as suggested by Guilfoyle & Noonan, 1988: 40: cf. Katz & Postal, 1964 and Grimshaw, 1993a, 1993b for arguments that adult English root yes-no involve a null counterpart of *whether*).

However, if we posit that at a later stage, the subject raises to spec-IP (and consequently carries nominative case), then we should expect (at this second phase of the IP/VP stage) to find that wh-phrases can no longer move to spec-IP (since this is now filled by the nominative subject), and instead adjoin to IP (as suggested by Guilfoyle & Noonan, 1988:40). Potential examples of this kind of structure include examples such as the following (from Klima & Bellugi, 1966: 205):

(56) Where the other Joe will drive? Where I should put it when I make up? What he can ride in? Why he don't know how to pretend? Why kitty can't stand up? How he can be a doctor? How they can't talk? Which way they should go?

Just as wh-phrases adjoin to VP when they immediately precede oblique subjects but to IP when they immediately precede nominative subjects, so too it seems that topic phrases can be adjoined either to the left of a VP with an oblique subject, or to the left of an IP with a nominative subject: cf.

(57) A train *me* got. A car *me* got (Nina 2;5, file 30)
     My tights *I* want (Nina 2;5, file 30)

Thus, there seems to be parallelism between the syntax of topics and the syntax of wh-phrases at this point.

At around two and a half years of age, children begin to acquire a COMP projection — as is suggested by the fact that they begin to use overt complementisers: cf.

(58) See *if* swimming water's there (Jem 2;3)
     You know *that* the flute is in there (Hannah 2;7)
     Leave a little space *for* them to get out (Helen 2;7)

At this point, they enter a third (CP) stage in their acquisition of clause structure, and an additional potential landing-site for wh-phrases becomes available — namely spec-CP. If wh-phrases move to spec-CP, we expect to find that auxiliaries move from INFL to COMP (in order to satisfy the requirement that heads be filled), and that the subject will raise from spec-VP to spec-IP and carry nominative case, so resulting in adult-like structures such as:

(59) What's he doing? What's he do? (Eve 2;0, file 13)
     How did he get out? (Nina 2;9, file 32)
     Why can't we open this piano? (Nina 2;9, file 33)
     Can I have it? Can I do that? Shall I close it? Are we going on an aeroplane now? What's she doing? What's she saying? What's he got? Why was he gone? (Heather 2;2)

Jill de Villiers (1991) argues that there is a significant correlation between the point at which children acquire embedded questions containing a given wh-item and the point at which they acquire root inversion questions with the same wh-item (e.g. a correlation between the emergence of embedded *what?* questions and root *what*+Auxiliary+ Subject questions). Why should this be?

One likely answer is that embedded wh-questions 'force' the child to posit an additional functional projection. The reason is that UG principles (cf. Chomsky, 1986) ban adjunction to arguments (i.e. to selected complements of lexical heads), so that the child 'knows' that embedded wh-questions cannot involve wh-adjunction to IP. Once the child has acquired CP (and comes to 'realise' that all finite complement clauses are CPs), the child concludes that that wh-phrases in embedded clauses move to spec-CP; given that UG principles prohibit movement into the head position of a lexically selected complement (cf. Rizzi & Roberts, 1989), the child will 'know' that auxiliaries cannot move from INFL to COMP in embedded questions, so that there will be no auxiliary inversion in embedded questions.[25] It seems reasonable to suppose that the child further assumes that if spec-CP is the landing-site for preposed wh-phrases in embedded clauses, spec-CP will also be available as a landing-site for preposed wh-phrases in root clauses as well. In the case of a root wh-question, spec-CP will then be filled by a preposed wh-phrase and the head COMP position will be filled by moving an auxiliary from INFL to COMP (in order to satisfy the requirement that non-selected heads be filled), so resulting in 'wh-inversion' structures like (59).

Independent evidence of aux-movement from INFL to COMP in root interrogative clauses at this later (CP) stage comes from the phenomenon of *auxiliary copying*, illustrated by the following examples (from Davis, 1987, cited in Roeper, 1991):

(60) What's he's doing? What's the mouse *is* doing? Why *is* there's big tears? What *is* the woman *is* doing? *Is* Tom *is* busy? *Is* it's Stan's radio? *Is* this *is* the powder? *Is* that's a belt?

If we assume that *copying* is a process by which both links in the relevant movement chain are lexicalised, it is reasonable to conclude that structures such as (60) provide us with evidence of aux-movement to COMP (and hence of a CP projection).

Suppose that we make the following additional set of assumptions:

(61) (i)   Children have to (lexically) learn the landing-site for specific types of wh-constituent (once they start to produce a given type of wh-constituent in embedded questions with uninverted auxiliaries, we have evidence that they have identified spec-CP as a licit landing-site for the relevant type of wh-constituent)

(ii)   Children learn the syntax (e.g. landing-site) of different types of wh-constituent at different stages of development (e.g. the syntax of *what*? questions is mastered before the syntax of *why*? questions)

(iii)   When they first acquire a given type of functional extended projection, children initially only *optionally* project the relevant functional architecture (cf. (49) above).

The claim in (61)(i) is supported by the fact that wh-landing sites vary parametrically from one language to another, and from one type of constituent to another (e.g. wh-adjuncts may adjoin to IP in Spanish, but wh-arguments move to spec-IP); the remark in parentheses in (61)(i) is supported by the findings reported in de Villiers (1991).

The set of assumptions in (61) may help us begin to account for the complex set of lexical effects which Labov & Labov (1978) report in their daughter Jessie's acquisition of auxiliary inversion in wh-questions. From the graph which they present on page 23 of their article, it would appear that when Jessie was 3;8, she showed obligatory use of auxiliary inversion in *how* questions, no use of inversion in *why?* questions, and sporadic use of inversion in *where?* (around 45%) and *what* (around 25%) questions. How can we explain this inversion asymmetry between the different types of wh-question?

Obligatory inversion after *how?* would indicate that Jessie at the relevant stage had identified spec-CP as the (unique) landing-site for *how?* The total absence of inversion after *why?* would indicate that she had not yet identified spec-CP as a licit landing-site for *why?*, and simply adjoined *why* to IP (with the *Minimal Projection Principle* ensuring that the clause would not further project into a vacuous CP). Optional inversion after *where/what?* would suggest that spec-CP had been identified as a possible landing-site for *where/what?*, but the optionality of inversion suggests that IP-adjunct position remained an alternative landing site (again, with the clause projecting no further than IP in such cases). What all of this tells us is that there is a strong component of *lexical learning* involved in the acquisition of wh-questions. Only when the child has learned that spec-CP is the *only* licit S-structure position for moved interrogative wh-phrases in English can we say that the full adult clause structure has been acquired.

9. Summary and Conclusion

In section 1, I provided a brief outline of SCH, and of the criticisms which have been levelled at it. In subsequent sections, I attempted to show that SCH provides a more satisfactory account of numerous characteristics of CICs than alternative functional analyses. In section 2, I argued that SCH can provide a principled account of null subjects in (declarative and interrogative) CICs if we assume (with Rizzi and Hyams) that null subjects can be discourse-identified in root positions. In section 3, I argued that the fact that children's early root clauses are nonfinite can similarly be accounted for if we posit that nonfinite verbs escape tense-binding requirements in root positions. In section 4, I suggested that subjects might be assigned inherent case, structural case or default case. In sections 5 and 6, I argued that early negative and interrogative sentences typically involve adjunction of the negative/interrogative constituent to VP, and that the S-structure location of the negative or interrogative constituent is determined by UG principles relating to *scope* and *minimal projection*. In section 7, I argued that there is empirical evidence for a Small Clause stage in other child languages, but that we cannot exclude the possibility that the SC stage might be 'silent' for (at least some) children acquiring languages with a rich verbal morphosyntax. In section 8, I looked at the inter-related questions of why early child clauses are VPs (highlighting the possible role of lexical, structural and maturational factors), and how children subsequently develop IP and CP projections. I suggested a three-stage VP>IP>CP model in which functional architecture is acquired 'one layer at a time', but is initially optionally projected (so that at stage I clauses are VPs, at stage II they are VPs or IPs, and at stage III they are VPs, IPs or CPs). In the case of wh-questions, such an analysis predicts (*inter alia*) that as clauses 'grow bigger', wh-complements of ergative verbs will come to occupy ever higher positions within the clause: e.g. in *Where go train?*, where is in spec-VP; in *Where train go?* it is in adj-VP; in *Where will train go?* it is in spec-IP; in *Where the train will go?* it is in adj-IP; and in *Where will the train go?*, it is in spec-CP. Thus, the SC analysis provides an intuitively plausible model in which children pass from an initial stage when they form only simple projections to subsequent stages in which they come to form ever more complex extended projections.

Notes

1. I am grateful to Harald Clahsen for helpful comments on an earlier version of this paper.
2. I maintain that the 'Small Clause' stage precedes Wexler's (1994) *optional infinitive* stage and Rizzi's (1993) *optional functional projections* stage, since at the stage Wexler and Rizzi are talking about, children alternate between finite and nonfinite root clauses.
3. Alongside verbal small clauses such as those in (1–3) above, children also produce verbless small clauses such as those in (i) below, which seem to be counterparts of adult verbal clauses headed by the copula be: cf.

(i) Wayne in bedroom (Daniel 1;9)
   Hand cold. Fire hot (Elen 1;8)
   Sausage bit hot (Jem 1;11)

   If we adopt the hypothesis put forward in Grimshaw (1991) that all clauses are projections of a head lexical verb, it follows that principles of UG require us to posit that such clauses are headed by an abstract (e.g.) copular verb: and indeed, this is the 'standard' position which has been adopted in relation to the analysis of verbless clauses in adult languages (cf. Fassi-Fehri 1993 on Arabic verbless clauses).
4. Throughout this paper, I have assumed that subjects originate in spec-VP, following the VP-internal subjects hypothesis suggested for adult grammars in for example Kitagawa, 1986; Kuroda, 1988; Sportiche, 1988; Diesing, 1990 and Koopman & Sportiche, 1991 — and indeed Hyams herself (p. 39) makes a parallel assumption in relation to her discussion of Icelandic. This assumption does not affect any of the arguments presented in this chapter.
5. Unless we assume that wh-phrases which move at LF for scope reasons adjoin to CP; or unless we posit that in adult null-subject sentences such as *Why bother?*, *why* is a CP-adjunct.
6. The analysis in the text accounts only for null subjects. As has been noted by P. Bloom (1990), English children also make sporadic use of null objects. One way of accounting for null objects would be to suppose that they involve topicalisation, e.g. a null topic adjoined to VP which binds an empty category of some kind in object position. Since the null topic would be in a root (VP-adjunct) position, it could be discourse-identified. If we assume (following

Hyams & Wexler, 1993: 431) that topicalisation is infrequent in early child English (as indeed it is in adult English), we then have a natural account of the relative scarcity of null objects in CICs.

7. Or by an untensed constituent which is itself tense-bound. For example, in a sentence like *He seems to be happy*, *be* is bound by the untensed infinitive particle *to* which in turn is bound by the tensed verb *seems*.

8. An alternative way of dealing with the root nonfinite verbs produced by young children would be to suppose that they are covertly tensed. For example, if we follow Halle & Marantz (1993) in positing that +*ing* is a present participle affix and that +*n* is a past participle affix in adult English, we might conjecture that children are initially unaware of the distinction between participles and finite verb forms, and so treat (e.g.) *going* as a present tense form and *gone* as a past tense form. An analysis along these lines has been proposed by Nina Hyams, who claims (1992b: 395, fn 8) that 'English speaking children mark finiteness by means of the progressive', cf. also her (1994: 44) remark that 'the real present tense affix is +*ing* which is acquired relatively early.' However, analysing participles as tensed verb forms still leaves the problem of how infinitive forms like *go* are to be analysed. Moreover, such an analysis presupposes that Negation is initially generated above Tense in child sentences such as 'No Mommy going/gone shops' — an assumption which makes for obvious discontinuity with adult English, where the converse hierarchical ordering holds. An additional problem is that early child clauses often have oblique subjects — not the nominative subjects which the 'tensed participles' analysis would lead us to expect, given that *tensed* forms license nominative specifiers (cf. Watanabe, 1993). A final problem worth noting is that the assumption that participles are finite forms raises the question of how children delearn their miscategorisation of them as tensed forms.

   The analysis proposed in the text accounts for the observation made by Plunkett (1991: 137, fn.13) that young children frequently omit *be* in root (but not embedded) wh-questions. If we assume that finite verbs are not tense-bound, an embedded finite V cannot have its tense properties determined by tense-binding, nor from discourse (since it is not in a root position): hence, it cannot be null. More generally, we predict that the only finite clauses which can be auxiliariless are root clauses. Finite root clauses with a null auxiliary persist for a considerable time, cf. Radford (1992b, 1992c). Note also that adult auxiliariless root clauses such as 'Where you been?' are amenable to a similar discourse-determined-tense analysis.

9. Of course, it is perfectly true that in Portuguese inflected infinitives, a nonfinite INFL licenses a nominative subject (Raposo, 1987). However, the important difference is that Portuguese infinitives are inflected for agreement — but English infinitives are not.

10. Vainikka (1993) reports that the earliest recorded clausal structures produced by Eve and Sarah typically have nominative subjects. However (as Vainikka herself notes), we should not exclude the possibility that nominative subjects herald the development of IP structures. This might mean that a child who alternates between *Me/I want cookie* has entered the stage where IP is optionally projected, and that *Me want cookie* is a VP structure, and *I want cookie* is an IP structure.

11. The discussion in this section of the text is based on the premise that early child (pro)nominals carry case. However, it should be pointed out that Radford (1986), Lebeaux (1988) and Kazman (1988) argued that there is no morphological marking of case in early child grammars, and concluded from this that *case* is not used as a syntactic licensing mechanism. Advocates of the strong continuity hypothesis counterargue that if we assume that the *visibility*

condition is a principle of UG which is operative in early child grammars, then nominals must indeed be assigned case (even if only abstractly) in order to be visible for theta-marking. Vainikka (1993) argues that the fact that even very young children have a contrast between (e.g.) *me* and *my* requires us to posit the existence of morphological case. However, the argument is potentially problematic, given that *my* might be analysed as a determiner rather than a genitive form of *me*: a determiner analysis would account for obvious asymmetries such as 'This is *John's/*my*'. For children who use *my* as the subject of a verb, a genitive case analysis seems more plausible. The argument in the text is overall of the form 'Even if we do assume the existence of syntactic case in early child grammars, SCH provides a more plausible account of the relevant facts than functional analyses.'

12. ECM structures seem to be productive in early child grammars: for example, Vainikka (1993: 46) notes that 'Adam produces this construction 75 times in 7 files between ages 2;6 and 2;9, using the main verbs *let, see* and *want*.'

13. Nina Hyams (1994: 28, ex. 9) offers a slightly different analysis in which the negative *no(t)* occupies the head NEG position of NEGP. In general, the observations made about Pierce's analysis in the text carry over to Hyams' analysis.

14. The *Minimal Projection Principle* is related to a number of conditions proposed in the literature. These include Chomsky's (1988) *Economy of Representation* principle, Grimshaw's (1993a, 1993b) *Minimal Projection* principle, and the principle of *Economy of Projection* proposed in Speas (1994).

15. These are generally considered to be 'routines' (Pierce, 1989: 86; Radford, 1990: 124–29; Plunkett, 1991: 134; Vainikka, 1993: 19). A number of linguists have argued that '*s* in early copula structures questions is mis-segmented by the child as part of the subject pronoun (cf. Bellugi, 1967; Brown, 1973; Bowerman, 1982; Peters, 1983; Hyams, 1992b:391). Vainikka (1993) suggests that '*s* may be a marker of the genitive case assigned to the subjects of Small Clauses by some children. For an alternative view, see notes 17 and 22.

16. The only other wh-question of the relevant type produced by Claire at age 24 months is 'What happen?': in this case, *what* might be the subject of *happen*, or might a preposed ergative complement. Given uncertainty about how to analyse this sentence, I have excluded it from the discussion here.

17. It may be that questions like 'What happen?' (cf. note 16) are ergative structures in which the subject originates in comp-VP and moves to spec-VP. It may even be that so-called 'routine questions' like 'What's that?' are also ergative structures, with the subject *that* in comp-VP, and the wh-phrase *what* in spec-VP. A VP-adjunction analysis of early wh-movement in nonergative clauses is proposed (e.g.) in Guilfoyle and Noonan, 1988: 37; Radford, 1990: 134 and Vainikka, 1993: 20, 25, 33. The precise nature of the empty category bound by the wh-phrase in early wh-questions produced by children is unclear. It may be a null resumptive pronoun (as suggested by Roeper *et al.*, 1985 and Nishigauchi & Roeper, 1987), or a null constant (cf. Roeper & de Villiers, 1992, and Vainikka & Roeper, 1993: 2. fn 3), or a variable.

18. It should be noted, however, that the children studied by Echeverría were more than two years old, and arguably well past the SC stage. Hernández Pina (1984) does not report early CVS structures — though does report early CV structures which might taken to be CVS structures with null subjects (but could equally be interpreted in many other ways, e.g. Tsimpli (1992) argues that such structures are VPs in which the complement can either precede or follow the verb within V-bar).

19. All the more so if we posit that there is initially no fixed linear ordering of complements with respect to their verbs, or of subjects with respect to V-bar: CVS structures would then be simple VPs in which the complement precedes

the verb, and the subject follows V-bar (cf. Tsimpli (1992) for an analysis along these lines).

20. Note, however, that the structural account does not in principle exclude the possibility that (say) VP and IP might be acquired simultaneously. In other words, the account excludes the possibility of IP being acquired before VP, but allows for the twin possibilities that either VP is acquired before IP, or IP is acquired at the same time as VP. We might therefore expect that whereas some children have a clearcut VP stage (preceding the IP stage), others do not. This could account for why studies of different children acquiring the same language lead different researchers to different conclusions (some arguing that children have VPs at stage I, others arguing that they have IPs, others that they have CPs).

21. Whether or not the first extended projection of V is IP is more problematic. An interesting problem in this regard is posed by the observation in Bowerman (1973) that Kendall initially used not only SVC order but also CVS order. In Radford (1990: 248–50), I suggested that Kendalls' CVS sentences are simple projections with noncanonical projection of the complement into spec-VP (for discourse reasons). However, another possibility is that CVS structures like *Mommy hit Kendall* are extended projections which involve raising the verb into a superordinate head position (designated as X below), and the complement into a superordinate specifier position, as in (i) below:

(i) $[_{XP}$ Complement$_i$ $[_X$ Verb$_j]$ $[_{VP}$ Subject $[_V$ e$_j]$ e$_i]]$

X might be a categorially un(der)specified head at this stage, so that XP is a 'shell' which is projected purely to enable focusing of the complement, cf. the discussion of (48) in the main text. It could be that (i) is the precursor of later IP structures, and that subsequently X is restricted to containing auxiliaries, and spec-XP is restricted to subjects. If (i) is the appropriate analysis of Kendall's CVS structures, it would seem that in some ways Kendall's grammar at the relevant stage of development is closer to that of adult German than to that of adult English .

22. One possibility which this raises is that early copular structures such as *That's Daddy car*, *There's Mummy*, *What's that?* and *Where's Teddy?* are not 'formulaic' utterances at all, but rather are early IP structures in which *be* is in INFL (perhaps tense-binding a null verb in V), and the preverbal constituent is in spec-IP. This in turn raises the possibility that early verbless questions like *What that?* may be IPs headed by a null copula in INFL, rather than 'formulaic' utterances. Such an analysis seems plausible for sentences such as *What dat for?* produced by Adam at 2;4. As noted in footnote 8, the analysis in the text would predict that children use null copulas in root positions — but not in embedded clauses.

23. The suggestion that early wh-questions involve wh-movement to spec-IP is found in Plunkett (1992: 73); Déprez and Pierce (1993: 59) and Vainikka (1993: 38).

24. Vainikka reports Nina (2;1, file 10) saying *There was monkeys*. Presumably we have a related case of spec-head agreement within IP here, with expletive *there* carrying the default person/number specification 3SG, and hence co-occurring with the 3SG verb form *was*.

25. Sporadic examples of inversion in embedded wh-questions are reported in the literature (cf.Plunkett, 1991: 131 and the following examples from Stromswold, 1990, cited by Déprez & Pierce, 1993: 59):

(i) I don't know who is dat. I don't know what is his name. I don't know what do you think it was. I don't know what is that bunny called. I don't know what ingredient do you use to make gumdrops. I don't know what's that.

For the reasons given in the text, these cannot involve wh-movement to spec-CP and aux-movement to C. Rather, they must be examples of IP questions in which the wh-phrase moves to spec-IP and the auxiliary is base-generated in INFL — and indeed, this is what Déprez and Pierce claim.

References

Abney, S.P. (1987) *The English Noun Phrase in its Sentential Aspect*. PhD dissertation, MIT.

Adone-Resch, M.C.D. (1990) *The Acquisition of Mauritian Creole as a First Language*. Ph.D dissertation, University of Düsseldorf.

Adone, M.C.D. (1993) 'IP and its development in Mauritian Creole', draft manuscript, University of Hamburg.

Akmajian, A. (1984) Sentence types and the form-function fit, *Natural Language and Linguistic Theory*, 2: 1–23.

Aldridge, M. (1989) *The Acquisition of INFL*, monograph, Indiana University Linguistics Club Publications, Bloomington Indiana.

Bellugi, U. (1967) *The Acquisition of Negation*. Ph.D dissertation, Harvard.

Bloom, L. (1970) *Language Development*. Cambridge, MA: MIT Press.

—. (1973) *One Word at aTime*. The Hague: Mouton.

Bloom, P. (1990) Subjectless sentences in child language: *Linguistic Inquiry* 21: 491–504

Bowerman, M. (1973) *Early Syntactic Development*, Cambridge University Press.

—. (1982) Reorganisational processes in lexical and syntactic development. In E. Wanner and L. Gleitman (eds) *Language Acquisition: The State of the Art*. Cambridge University Press. 319–46.

Bresnan, J.W. (1976) On the form and functioning of transformations, *Linguistic Inquiry* 7: 3–40.

Brown, R. (1973) *A First Language: The Early Stages*. London: George Allen and Unwin.

Budwig, N. (1984) Me, My and Name: Children's Early Systematizations of Forms, Meanings and   Functions in Talk about the Self, draft manuscript, University of California, Berkeley; *Papers and Reports on Child Development*, 24.

— (1985) The expression of transitivity by a 2-year-old child. In W. Kürschner, R. Vogt & S. Siebert-Nemann (eds) *Sprachtheorie, Pragmatik. Interdisziplinäres*, Tübingen: Niemeyer. pp. 291–302.

— (1989) The linguistic marking of agentivity and control in child language, *Journal of Child Language* 16: 263–84.

Chiat, S. (1981) Context-specificity and generalisations in the acquisition of pronominal distinctions, *Journal of Child Language* 8, 75–91.

Chomsky, N. (1973) Conditions on transformations In S.R. Anderson and P. Kiparsky (eds) *A Festschrift for Morris Halle*. New York: Holt Rinehart and Winston. pp. 232–86.

— (1986) *Barriers*. Cambridge, MA: MIT Press.

— (1988) Some notes on economy of derivation and representation, draft manuscript, MIT.

Cinque, G. (1988) Parameter-setting in 'instantaneous' and 'real-time' acquisition. *Behavioural and Brain Sciences* 12, 336–7.

Clark, E.V. (1985) The acquisition of Romance with special reference to French. In D.I. Slobin, (ed) *The Crosslinguistic Study of Language Acquisition, 1*, (pp. 687–780).

Davis, H. (1987) *The Acquisition of the English Auxiliary System and its relation to Linguistic Theory*, Ph.D dissertation, University of British Columbia.

Déprez, V. and Pierce, A. (1993) Negation and functional projections in early grammar, *Linguistic Inquiry* 24 : 47–85.

— (1994) Crosslinguistic evidence for functional projections in early child grammar. In T. Hoekstra & B.D. Schwartz (eds), *Language Acquisition in Generative Grammar*. Amsterdam: Benjamins. pp. 57–84.

de Villiers, J. (1991) Why questions? In T.L. Maxfield & B. Plunkett (eds), *Papers in the Acquisition of WH*. Amherst: GLSA Publiciations. pp. 155–73.

Diesing, M. (1990) Verb movement and the subject position in Yiddish, *Natural Language and Linguistic Theory* 8: 41–79.

Echeverría, M.D. (1978) *Dearrollo de la comprensión de la sintaxis española*, Serie Lingüistica 3, University of Concepción, Chile.

Fassi-Fehri, A. (1993) *Issues in the structure of Arabic Clauses and Words*, Dordrecht: Kluwer.

Gawlitzek-Maiwald, I., Tracy, R. and Fritzenschaft, A. (1992) Language acquisition and competing linguistic representations: The child as arbiter. In J. Meisel (ed). *The Acquisition of Verb Placement: Functional Categories and V2 Phonemena in Language Acquisition*. Dordrecht: Kluwer. pp. 139–79.

Gleitman, L. and Wanner, E. (1982) Language acquisition: the state of the state of the art. In E. Wanner and L. Gleitman (eds). *Language Acquisition: The State of the Art*. Cambridge University Press. pp. 3–48.

Grimshaw, J. (1991) Extended Projection, draft manuscript, Brandeis University, July 1991.

— (1993a) Minimal Projection, Heads, and Optimality, draft manuscript, Rutgers University, June 1993.

— (1993a) Minimal Projection, Heads, and Optimality, conference handout, Rutgers University, November 1993 [revised version of Grimshaw 1993a].

Gruber, J. (1967) Topicalisation in child language, *Foundations of Language* 3: 37–65.

Guasti, M. T. (1992) Verb syntax in Italian child grammar, *Geneva Generative Papers*, vol 0, no. 2, pp. 145–62.

Guilfoyle, E. and Noonan, M. (1988) Functional categories and language acquisition, text of paper presented at the 13th Annual Boston University conference on Language Development, Boston, 13th October.

Halle, M. and Marantz, A. (1993) Distributed morphology and the pieces of inflection. In K. Hale, & S.J. Keyser, (eds) *The View from Building 20*. MIT Press, pp. 111–76.

Hernández Pina, R. (1984) *Teorías Psico-Sociolinqüísticas y su Aplicación a la adquisición del Español como Lenqua Materna*, Siglo XXI, Madrid.

Hill, J.A.C. (1983) *A Computational Model of Language Acquisition in the Two Year-Old*. Indiana University Linguistics club, Bloomington, Indiana.

Hoekstra, T. and Jordens, P. (1994) From adjunct to head. In T. Hoekstra & B.D. Schwartz (eds). *Language Acquisition Studies in Generahve Grammar*. Amsterdam: Benjamins. pp. 119–49.

Huxley, R. (1970) The development of the correct use of subject pronouns in two children. In G. Flores d'Arcais and W. Levelt (eds) *Advances in Psycholinguistics*. Amsterdam: North Holland. pp . 141–65.

Hyams, N. (1986) *Language Acquisition and the Theory of Parameters*, Dordrecht: Reidel.

— (1992) The genesis of clausal structure. In J. Meisel (ed). *The Acquisition of Verb Placement: Functional Categories and V2 Phenomena in Language Acquisition*. Dordrecht: Kluwer. pp. 371–400.

— (1994) V2, null arguments and COMP projections. In T. Hoekstra & B.D. Schwartz (eds). *Language Acquisition Studies in Generative Grammar*. Amsterdam: Benjamins. pp. 21–55.

Hyams, N. and Wexler, K. (1993) On the grammatical basis of null subjects in child language, *Linguistic Inquiry* 24: 421–59.

Jackendoff, R. S. (1974) *Introduction to the $\bar{X}$ Convention*. Indiana University Linguistics Club.

— (1977) $\bar{X}$ *Syntax: A Study of Phrase Structure*. Cambridge, MA: MIT Press.

Jimenez, M.-L. Subject-verb inversion in Spanish, abstract of paper presented to LSA meeting, January 1994.

Katz, J.J. and Postal, P.M. (1964) *An Integrated Theory of Linguistic Descriptions*, Cambridge, MA: MIT Press.

Kazman, R. (1988) Null arguments and the acquisition of case and infl, draft manuscript, Carnegie Mellon University.

Kitagawa, Y. (1986) *Subjects in Japanese and English*, Ph.D diss., University of Massachusetts.

Klima, E.S. and Bellugi, U. (1966) Syntactic Regularities in the Speech of Children. In J. Lyons, & R. Wales,(eds) *Psycholinguistic Papers*. Edinburgh University Press, pp. 183–207.

Koopman, H. and Sportiche, D. (1991) The position of subjects, *Lingua* 18: 211–58.

Kraskow, T. (1994) Slavic multiple questions: Evidence for wh-movement, abstract of paper presented to LSA meeting, January 1994.

Kuroda, Y (1988) Whether we agree or not: a comparative syntax of English and Japanese, *Linguisticae Investigationes* 12: 1–47.

Labov, W. and Labov, T. 1978. Learning the syntax of questions. In R.N. Campbell, & P.T. Smith, (eds) *Recent Advances in the Psychology of Language*, New York: Plenum Press. pp. 1–54.

Lebeaux, D. (1987) Comments on Hyams. In T. Roeper & E. Williams (eds) *Parameter Setting*. pp. 23–39.

— (1988) *Language Acquisition and the Form of the Grammar*. PhD dissertation, University of Massachusetts.

McNeill, D. (1966) Developmental psycholinguistics. In F. Smith and G.A. Miller, (eds). *The Genesis of Language: a Psycholinguistic Approach*. Cambridge, MA: MIT Press. pp. 15–84.

Meisel, J. (1992) Getting FAT: Finiteness, Agreement and Tense in early grammars, draft manuscript, University of Hamburg to appear in J. Meisel (ed.) *Bilingual First Language Acquisition: French and German Grammatical Development*. Amsterdam: Benjamins.

Menyuk, P. (1969) *Sentences Children Use*, Cambridge, MA: MIT Press.

Nishigauchi, T. and Roeper, T. (1987) Deductive parameters and the growth of empty categories. In T. Roeper & E. Williams (eds). *Parameter Setting*. Dordrecht: Reidel. pp. 91–121.

Penner, Z. (1992) The ban on parameter resetting, default mechanisms, and the acquisition of V2 in Bernese Swiss German. In J. Meisel (ed). *The Acquisition of Verb Placement: Functional Categories and V2 Phenomena in Language Acquisition*. Dordrecht: Kluwer.

Peters, A. (1983) *The Units of Language Acquisition*. Cambridge University Press.

Phinney, M. (1981) *Syntactic Constraints and the Acquisition of Embedded Sentential Complements*. Ph.D dissertation, University of Massachusetts.

Pierce, A. (1989) *On the Emergence of Syntax: A Crosslinguistic Study*. Ph.D dissertation, MIT.

Platzack, C. (1990) A grammar without functional categories: A syntactic study of early Swedish child language, *Nordic Journal of Linguistics* 13: 107–26.

Plunkett, B. (1991) Inversion and early Wh questions. In T.L. Maxfield & B. Plunkett (eds). *Papers in the Acquisition of WH*. Amherst: GLSA Publications. pp. 125–53.

— (1992) Continuity and the landing site for Wh movement, *Bangor Research Papers in Linguistics* 4: 53–77.

Poeppel, D. and Wexler, K. (1993) The full competence hypothesis of clause structure in early German, *Language* 69:1, 1–33.

Radford, A. (1986) Small children's small clauses, *Bangor Research Papers in Linguistics* 1: 1–38.

— (1990) *Syntactic Theory and the Acquisition of English Syntax*, Oxford:Blackwell.
— (1992a) Comments on Roeper and de Villiers In J. Weissenborn, H. Goodluck & T. Roeper (eds). *Theoretical Issues in Language Acquisition*. Hillsdale, NJ: Erlbaum. pp. 237–48.
— (1992b) The acquisition of the morphosyntax of finite verbs in English In J.M. Meisel (ed) *The Acquisition of Verb Placement*, Dordrecht: Kluwer. pp. 23–62.
— (1992c) Tense and agreement variability in child grammars, text of paper presented to the symposium on *Syntactic Theory and First Language Acquisition*, Cornell University.
— (1993) Head-hunting: on the trail of the nominal Janus, In G. Corbett *et al.* (eds) *Heads in Grammatical Theory*. Cambridge University Press, pp. 73–113.
— (1994) The morphosyntax of subjects and verbs in child Spanish: A case study, paper presented to the Symposium on the Acquisition of Case and Agreement, University of Essex. March 1994.
Radford, A. and Aldridge, M. (1987) The acquisition of the inflection system. In W. Lörscher & R. Schulze (eds) *Perspectives in Language in Performance*, Narr, Tübingen, vol 2, pp. 1289–1309.
Randall, J. H. (1992) The catapult hypothesis: An approach to unlearning. In J. Weissenborn, H. Goodluck and T. Roeper (eds). *Theoretical Issues in Language Acquisition*. Hillsdale, NJ: Erlbaum. pp. 93–138.
Raposo, E. (1987) Case theory and INFL-to-COMP: the inflected infinitive in European Portuguese, *Linguistic Inquiry* 18: 85–109.
Rizzi, L. (1992) Early null subjects & root null subjects, *Geneva Generative Papers*, vol 0, no. 2, pp. 102–14.
— (1993) Some notes on linguistic theory and language development, draft manuscript, University of Geneva.
— (1984) Early null subjects and root null subject. In T. Hoekstra and B.D. Schwartz (eds). *Language Acquisition Studies in Generative Grammar*. Amsterdam: Benjamins. pp. 151–76.
Rizzi, L. and Roberts, I. (1989) Complex Inversion in French, *Probus* 1:1–30.
Roeper, T. (1991) How a marked parameter is chosen: Adverbs and *do*-insertion in the IP of child grammar. In T. Maxfield and B. Plunkett (eds) *Papers in the Acquisition of WH*. Amherst: GLSA Publications. pp. 175–202.
— (1992) Acquisition principles in action. In J. Meisel (ed). *The Acquisition of Verb Placement: Functional Categories and V2 Phenomena in Language Acquisition*. Dordrecht: Kluwer. pp. 333–70.
Roeper, T., Akiyama, S., Mallis, L., and Rooth, M. (1985) The problem of empty categories and bound variables in language acquisition, unpublished manuscript, Univ. of Massachusetts.
Roeper, T. and de Villiers, J. (1991) Introduction: acquisition of Wh-movement. In T.I. Maxfield & B. Plunkett. *Papers in the Acquisition of WH*. Amherst: GLSA Publiciations. pp. 1–18.
— (1992a) Ordered decisions in the acquisition of Wh-questions. In J. Weissenborn, H. Goodluck & T. Roeper. *Theoretical Issues in Language Acquisition*. Hillsdale, NJ: Erlbaum. pp. 191–236.
Rudin, C. (1988) On multiple questions and multiple Wh fronting, *Natural Language and Linguistic Theory* 6: 445–501.
Solan, L. and Roeper, T. (1978) Children's use of syntactic structure in interpreting relative clauses. In *Papers in the Structure and Development of Child Language*, UMASS Occasional Papers in Linguistics, vol 4.
Speas, M. (1994) Null arguments in a theory of economy of projection, abstract of paper presented to Boston meeting of LSA, January 1994.
Sportiche, D. (1988) A theory of floating quantifiers, *Linguistic Inquiry* 19: 425–50.
Tsimpli, I . M. (1992) *Functional Categories and Maturation: The Prefunctional Stage of Language Acquisition*, Ph.D dissertation, University College London.

Vainikka, A. (1993) Case in the development of English syntax, draft manuscript, University of Pennsylvania.

Vainikka, A. and Roeper, T (1993) Abstract operators in early acquisition, draft manuscript, University of Massachusetts.

Watanabe, A. (1993) The notion of finite clauses in AGR-based case theory, *MIT Working Papers in Linguistics*, 18: 281–96.

Wexler, K (1994) Optional infinitives, head movement and the economy of derivations. In D. Lightfoot and N. Hornstein (eds) *Verb Movement* (pp.305–50). Cambridge: Cambridge University Press.

White, L. (1982) *Grammatical Theory and Language Acquisition*, Hingham, MA: Kluwer.

Williams, E. (1975) Small clauses in English. In J.P. Kimball (ed) *Syntax and Semantics* 4: 249–73.

Zagona, K. (1988) *Verb Phrase Syntax*. Dordrecht: Reidel.

Zanuttini, R. (1989) Two types of negative markers, *Proceedings of NELS 20*, GLSA, University of Massachusetts, Amherst.

12 Children's Attributions of Speakers' Pragmatic Intentions

KENNETH REEDER

This study's aims were to describe the types of intentions young school-aged children attribute to Speakers and their reported bases for such attributions, to describe metapragmatic knowledge involved, and to explore the extent to which children's accounts of their pragmatic comprehension were coherent and principled. Forty-one English-speaking children from 6;2 to 8;9 years were given a pragmatic paraphrase procedure designed to reveal illocutionary uptake. A subsequent interview was coded in terms of type of illocutionary intention attributed to the Speaker in the staged speech act, and the basis upon which subjects believed they had made that attribution. Findings revealed a good fit between speaker intentions and felicity conditions for illocutionary acts postulated. Children reported employing knowledge about cognition, social roles, proxemics, linguistic form, illocutionary acts, and pragmatic strategies including politeness conventions and maintenance of face.

What is the nature of school-age children's ability to attribute intentions to speakers in a conversational interaction? Speech Act theory (Searle, 1969, 1979) proposes two classes of felicity conditions which must be satisfied for the appropriate performance of a speech act: conditions pertaining to the propositional content of the utterance, and conditions pertaining to the participants in the discourse in question. In addition to interpreting features of the linguistic utterance, a conversationalist must attend to aspects of participants' knowledge, assumptions and attitudes in order to compute the illocutionary intent behind most everyday utterances and respond in some appropriate way, verbally or otherwise (Levinson, 1983: 1.4). In addition to linguistically-conveyed information about such participant features (henceforth, 'intentions'), extralinguistic cues will also be employed in the inferential process involved, particularly when little or no explicit information concerning illocutionary force is provided in the utterance itself, as in the case of polite indirect speech acts, ironic usage, and the like.

Studies of younger children's linguistic pragmatic abilities portray such children employing at least some degree of information about participants in a reliable way (Halliday, 1975; Shatz, 1978). The majority of those studies focus upon the extent to which young children take somewhat fixed features, such as age, status or role of speakers or hearers into account in formulating or responding to a speech act (Shatz & Gelman, 1973; James, 1975; Bates, 1976; Leonard & Reid, 1979; Becker, 1981; Ledbetter & Dent, 1988).

Somewhat later pragmatic studies included aspects of speakers which are more fortuitous such as intention or communicative goal in the scope of their investigation. Wilkinson, Wilkinson, Spinelli & Chiang (1984) found 5–8-year-olds quite exacting in terms of linguistic form when it came to accepting appropriate performances of requests for action, but less stringent for requests for information, implying that they took speakers' intentions into account when judging utterance appropriateness. Moreover, in their explanations of their judgements, not only speaker politeness but also the speaker's object in requesting was consistently mentioned by children across the age range studied.

Several recent studies focus upon such aspects of children's metapragmatic knowledge as politeness of directives (Baroni & Axia, 1989), politeness, effectiveness and likelihood of use (Garton & Pratt, 1990), strategic manipulations of communicative rule systems (Becker, 1988a), and responses to a particular class of parental efforts to teach pragmatic skills (Becker, 1988b).

In a study of 6 to 11-year-olds' ability to employ a speaker's general conversational goal in determining the point of an individual speech act, Abbeduto, Nuccio Bibler, Al-Mabuk, Rotto & Maas (1992) found that only the 11-year-olds and the adult controls were able to make the necessary semantic discriminations and consequently construct the preferred pragmatic responses, and concluded that only those age groups took speakers' goals into account when computing illocutionary point. A similar finding emerged from Bernicot & Laval's (1993) study of 4, 7 and 11-year-olds' understanding of felicity conditions of promises: only the 11-year-olds incorporated information about the speaker's intentions, or the joint intentions and desires of speaker and listener. However, earlier Reeder and Wakefield (1987) had shown three-year-olds reliably comprehending indirect requests even when linguistic information was systematically removed from the presentation, suggesting that even young children can make considerable use of contextual information. Hickmann, Champaud & Bassano (1993) studied 5 to 9-year-olds' pragmatic and metapragmatic knowledge of the rules of use for the French epistemic modal verb *croire* ('think', 'believe'). All age groups made use of the witnesses' epistemic status, i.e. their prior knowledge or lack thereof, in increasingly sophisticated ways.

Thus the extent and precise nature of children's ability to take participant information into account in conversational tasks remains at the least ill-defined, and to some extent, controversial. The primary aim of the present study was to describe the types of intentions young school-aged children attribute to Speakers, and to describe their reported bases for such attributions. A secondary aim was to add to our understanding of the extent to which such children could gain access to metapragmatic knowledge of their own comprehension processes in the linguistic pragmatic domain. A third aim was to explore the question of whether, and to what extent, the children's own accounts of their pragmatic comprehension were coherent and principled.

Method

Subjects

41 English-speaking children, 19 female and 22 male, from middle-class communities in two western Canadian cities took part in the study. Subjects ranged in age from 6;2 to 8;9 years, with a mean age of 7;2, and were attending grades one, two and three of local public and private schools where the language of instruction was predominantly English but in several cases, French. All children were judged by their teachers to possess native speaker proficiency in English, including several children for whom English was not the home language, and none exhibited discernible linguistic or learning difficulties or delays.

Procedure

Children were seen in quiet areas as close to their school classrooms as possible, and responses to the tasks audiotape-recorded for transcription later.

Paraphrases

The objective of this task was to elicit an illocutionary interpretation of a speaker's utterance. Presentations of the paraphrase task was by means of an audiotaped utterance ascribed to small figurines in a context found previously to predispose children to a directive interpretation. An adult puppet 'teacher' uttered a syntactically-scrambled version of the following to a puppet 'pupil':

(1) Would you like to (do) *A* ?

where *A* refers to participation in a playground scenario portrayed (e.g.

'play on the swings', 'ride the bike', etc.). This scenario, employing small-scale model playthings, is illustrated in Figure 12.1. The stimuli were degraded in each case in order to avoid strictly short-term memorized recounting which may have resulted in a ceiling effect. Following presentation of a stimulus item, the child was asked 'What was the teacher trying to say?' in order to elicit one attempted paraphrase, then 'What's another way to say that?' in order to elicit a second paraphrase response. We sought two paraphrase responses for each item per interview from subjects in view of the difficulty of inferring in an unambiguous way illocutionary force from linguistic form alone (Reeder, 1983). The second paraphrase for any item might corroborate or otherwise illuminate our initial analysis of how a child took up the utterance in question.

The scheme set out in Table 12.1 was constructed on the basis of the responses obtained, and the paraphrase responses then coded according to its categories by two coders, with disagreements resolved in each case by discussion. The two coders agreed initially in 84% of the cases, with the remainder reconciled as noted.

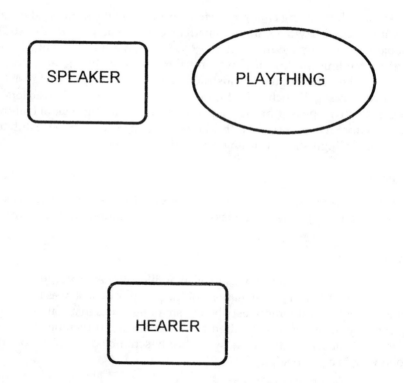

Figure 12.1 Predisposing context for paraphrase task.

Table 12.1 Coding scheme for paraphrases

Category	Example
Question	'Do you know how to make a picture?'
Request	'Please can you make a picture?'
Order	'You make a picture'
Suggestion	'Maybe you could draw a picture'
Offer	'You can make a picture'

Attribution of Speaker Intentions

Following elicitation of paraphrases, the interviewer asked the child 'Why do you think the teacher said that?' A taxonomy of response types shown in Table 12.2 was constructed on the basis of raw responses from these protocols. Speaker Intention responses were then coded according to that scheme by two coders whose initial codings agreed in 89% of cases, with disagreements of coding resolved by discussion.

Table 12.2 Coding scheme for attributions of speaker intentions

Category/Code	Example
Speaker wants A/S WANT A	'She wants them to draw a picture'
Speaker wants to know p/S KNOW P	'To find out if she could make a picture'
Speaker's role/S ROLE	'Because probably she's the art teacher and she would like the little girl to make a picture'
Hearer wants A/H WANT A	'The little kid was wondering if he could make a picture'
Hearer's role/H ROLE	'She didn't know how. She has to learn'
Institutional routines/ INSTITNL	'That's what you're supposed to do at school'

Basis for Attribution of Speaker Intentions

Once a response was elicited for the attribution probe, the interviewer asked 'How do you know that?' Tentative or unclear responses were probed further if necessary in an attempt to elicit a clear statement of subjects' bases for their attributions of intentionality to Speakers. A taxonomy of response types was constructed from the interview data, in an attempt to construct an exhaustive coding scheme for the data set as in

Table 12.3 Basis for subjects' attributions of speaker intentions coding scheme

Category/Code	Examples
Cognition/COGN	'I looked at it and I just thought'
Role knowledge/ROLE KN	'Well, if you're in school it's good to learn how to draw'
Proxemic/kinesic cue/ PROXEMIC	'Because she had the table right beside her'
Locutionary act/LOCUTION	'Well, she asked her so she probably means it'
Formal linguistic cue/FORM	'The way she uses her voice it seems like she wants the student to go there'
Illocutionary act, process/ ILLOC	'Because she asked a question, if he could make a picture'
Pragmatic strategy/PRAG	'The little girl probably doesn't like Art, and the Art teacher is saying 'please' because she wants her to'

Table 12.3. Responses were then coded in terms of its categories by two coders, with disagreements resolved by discussion in each case.

Results

Paraphrases

Results of the coding exercise for the paraphrase responses are presented in Table 12.4. The vast majority of children's paraphrase responses were coded as one or another category of illocutionary acts generally termed 'directives' (Searle, 1979) in the sense that there is some obligation placed upon the Hearer in such cases to respond with action or information.

The extent of the directive intent might be seen to vary along a scale from direct order at one end to suggestion at the other, least direct end. Even the offer paraphrases are linked pragmatically, in common with the more obviously directive categories, to some obligation of response on the Hearer's part, either to take up or reject the offer of the act predicated in the utterance.

Table 12.4 Categorization of paraphrases of stimulus utterance

Category	Trial 1		Trial 2		1 + 2 combined	
	N	%	N	%	N	%
Question	13	30.23	15	36.59	28	33.33
Request	16	37.21	22	53.66	38	45.24
Order	7	16.28	1	2.44	8	9.52
Suggestion	6	13.95	1	2.44	7	8.33
Offer	1	2.33	2	4.88	3	3.57
TOTAL	43	100	41	100	84	100

Attribution Probes

Qualitative analysis of the protocols in response to the question 'Why do you think the teacher said that?' together with any followup probes is summarized in Table 12.5.

Table 12.5 Attributions of speaker's intentions

Category*	Trial 1		Trial 2		1 + 2 combined	
	N	%	N	%	N	%
S WANTS A	26	52.00	20	47.62	46	50.00
S KNOWS P	13	26.00	10	23.81	23	25.00
S ROLE	4	8.00	2	4.76	6	6.52
H WANTS A	1	2.00	3	7.14	4	4.35
H ROLE	1	2.00	1	2.38	2	2.17
INSTITNL	5	10.00	6	14.29	11	11.96
TOTAL	50	100	42	100	92	100

* See Table 12.2 for glosses and examples of category codes.

Regardless of illocutionary uptake, children would often phrase their attributions of Speaker intention by referring to a felicity condition for the perceived illocutionary act. Additional evidence mentioned in the Speaker intention attributions included social role, or institutional routines. We then considered the question of whether the children's attributions were linked in some principled way to the particular speech acts they understood Speakers to have performed. This was done by means of a simple cross-tabulation of children's individual attributions with that trial's postulated speech act as shown in Table 12.6.

Table 12.6 Cross-tabulation of S intention responses by speech act paraphrase response category

Category	S Want A		S Know P		S Role		H Want A		H Role		Institnl	
	N	%	N	%	N	%	N	%	N	%	N	%
Question	5	10.87	18	78.26	1	16.67	3	75.00	1	50.00	1	9.0
Request	29	63.04	1	4.35	4	66.67	0	0	1	50.00	5	45.4
Order	6	13.04	1	4.35	1	16.67	0	0	0	0	2	18.1
Suggestion	5	10.87		8.70	0	0	0	0	0	0	2	18.1
Offer	1	2.17	1	4.35	0	0	1	25.00	0	0	1	9.0
TOTAL	46	100	23	100	6	100	4	100	2	100	11	100

The most frequently postulated basis for S's utterance was S Wants A, or some indication that the teacher wanted the pupil to do the act A mentioned in the predicate of the stimulus form. Examples ranged from the fairly direct statement in (2) to the more elaborate stratagem attributed to S in (3)

(2)   She wants them to draw a picture.

(3)   The teacher probably doesn't want them bothering her so she makes them go to the play area.

Table 12.6 indicates that S Wants A was associated with a Request speech act in 29 of the 46 cases. This is not surprising if we note that S Wants A is one of the essential felicity conditions upon a request, according to speech act theory. Moreover, a further 11 cases of S Wants A are associated with Order and Suggestion speech acts combined, both cases where S Wants A would constitute necessary conditions in the interpersonal context. Thus, in approximately 87% of the instances where S Wants A is postulated as a motive for the speech act, it is linked to a pragmatically appropriate speech act rather than to many of the other available but pragmatically-inappropriate speech act categories such as Question or Offer.

The next most frequently-attributed basis — 23 of the 92 cases, or 25% — for the stimulus utterance was S Know P, in the sense that the teacher wanted to know whether the pupil wanted to undertake the activity predicated, as in (4):

(4)   To find out if she could make a picture.

S Know P was associated with a Question speech act paraphrase in the vast majority of instances of this attribution of intent, just over 78% of the cases, with only one or two instances associated with each of the other speech act categories. Again, this is not surprising given that the most obvious felicity condition motivating an appropriately-performed question is the asker's interest in knowing P.

S's Role was employed in six of the 92 attributions, and was linked in four of those cases to Request paraphrases, as shown in (5):

(5) Because probably she's the Art teacher and she would like the little girl to make a picture.

The link with Request paraphrases in the majority of cases is not surprising in view of the convention, mentioned to children during familiarization with the task materials, that the adult speaker was a primary school teacher, presumably charged by virtue of this role with the direction of activity in the playground or schoolroom scenario set out before our subjects.

Hearer Wants A was attributed in four cases only, and was associated in three of those cases to Question paraphrases of the stimulus utterance, and in one case to an Offer. The link is quite explicitly made in the latter case, where the attribution is as follows:

(6) The little kid was wondering if she could make a picture

which in turn followed from this subject's paraphrase of the teacher's utterance:

(7) You can make a picture.

Linked to Question paraphrases were these mentions of H Wants A:

(8) The little girl was wondering what to do or doesn't know what to do.

(9) The little boy might want to play with the blocks.

Another minor category was H's role, linked in its two instances to a Question in one case, and in the following instance, to a Request paraphrase:

(10) She didn't know how. She has to learn.

A more frequent attribution made use of institutional conventions of early school experience or adult–child relations in general, and accounted for 11 of the 92 attributions offered. While five of the eleven cases were associated with Request paraphrases, as in the case of

(11) Maybe because there are too many children at the other stations

the remaining six were about equally distributed across the other paraphrase categories employed. This case was associated, for example, with an Offer paraphrase:

(12) Because it was a game and you could play it.

This subject followed the above with a rationale to the effect that the children were offered this activity 'so they won't bother the teacher and so they can play' in what we hoped was not a widely-held view of the role of teachers and schools!

Basis for Attribution of Intentions

Qualitative analysis of the protocols in response to the question 'How do you know that?' together with any followup probes are summarized in Table 12.7.

Table 12.7 Reported basis for attribution of speaker's intentions

Category	Trial 1		Trial 2		1 + 2 combined	
	N	%	N	%	N	%
COGN	7	15.22	8	17.39	15	16.30
ROLE KN	5	10.87	8	17.39	13	14.13
PROX	7	15.22	4	8.70	11	11.96
LOCUTION	15	32.61	22	47.83	37	40.22
FORM	7	15.22	2	4.35	9	9.78
ILLOC	3	6.52	2	4.35	5	5.43
PRAG	2	4.35	0	0	2	2.17
TOTAL	46	100	46	100	92	100

* See Table 12.3 for glosses and examples of category codes

Children described a wide range of bases for their attributions of S and H intentions. These included cognitive reasons (knowing, guessing, suspecting), proxemic and kinesic cues in the predisposing context, appeals to personal experience of the Speaker's or Hearer's roles, reference to pragmatic politeness or face-maintaining conventions, and reference to an illocutionary category or a literal locution performed.

Almost exactly half of the responses made reference either to the fact of, or the linguistic form of, the performance of the stimulus utterance itself. The majority of such cases referred to the Locution performed by the Speaker in the role play presented, as in the following:

(13) By the words on the tape

Several cases offered evidence about the pragmatic basis upon which children appeared to have been reconstructing the actual locution:

(14) Because she said 'would you like to look at the blocks?'

(15) Because she said 'can you draw a picture?'

In addition to such outright quotations, a half-dozen instances imputed an intention to the speaker which made pragmatic sense of the utterance, by means of indirect quotation:

(16) Because she was asking her if she wants to do it.

At least two Locution responses referred to what we took to have been an apprehension of Grice's Maxim of Relevance (1975), as in:

(17) Well she asked her so she probably means it.

Close to 10% of the responses made reference to the linguistic form of the stimulus utterance, mainly in terms of some actual or imagined prosodic features. Examples of formal linguistic justifications included:

(18) I can sort of hear a voice coming through the scribbly voice.

(19) Because she was mixing the words up but I could tell.

Just over 16% of the bases reported by children pertained to what we coded as Cognitive bases: the subject's own processes of knowing, guessing, and the like, or some reference to an imputed cognitive state or process of the participants in the play scenario, as in:

(20) I looked at it and I just thought.

(21) I just knew.

Some of the more interesting and complex responses coded as Cognitive bases were double-coded with one of the more strictly linguistic categories. The following response was coded both as a Cognitive response because of its reference to the speaker's imputed interests and the hearer's wants, but also as a reference to an Illocutionary Act, based upon its reference to 'asking':

(22) **E**: How do you know that?
　　 S: Cuz she's interested.
　　 E: Who?
　　 S: The teacher.
　　 E: In what?
　　 S: In what the little girl wants to do.
　　 E: How can you tell that?
　　 S: If she wasn't, she wouldn't ask.

One of the more extended responses combined Cognitive categories like uncertainty with an account of a process of illocutionary uptake:

(23) **E**: How do you know that?
　　 S: Because if the teacher asked him to do it, well, I don't know for sure. But I don't know if the boy or girl would want to do it. But I don't know for sure if he will. But I think he would.
　　 E: Why?
　　 S: Because I think he would like drawing pictures.

E: But you were saying something about 'Cuz if the teacher asked him to do it'.
S: Then he has to do it.

Just over 14% of the justifications made reference to the role played in the interaction either by speaker or hearer. Most such responses mentioned the teacher's professional role in some fashion:

(24) Because she's a teacher and she's supposed to teach the kids.

Some responses made references to the pupil's role:

(25) Well, if you're in school it's good to learn how to draw, not just be able to print . . .

Just how sophisticated that knowledge of teacher and pupil roles could be was demonstrated in the following paraphrase response, attribution of intention, and explanation of its basis:

(26) E: What did the teacher say?
    S: Can you show me if you can make a picture?
    E: Why do you think the teacher said that?
    S: To see what he [child puppet] can do.
    E: How do you know that?
    S: Cuz that's what all my other teachers wanted me to do.

While we coded the initial paraphrase in (26) as a Request, its structure and content show that it is a peculiarly pedagogical one, a request for display of knowledge. This seemed to us to demonstrate how this child could apply to the present task a well-developed grasp of teachers' behaviour in role, and of one discourse convention of teaching.

So strong were the social cues for participant intentionality, apparently, that what seemed to us a rather more obvious cue, that of proxemics, was not as frequently mentioned as we had expected. Roughly 12% of the justifications mentioned this feature of the scenario, as set out in Figure 12.1 above, in which the Speaker/teacher puppet was set alongside one plaything or activity in particular. Several subjects noted this fact in providing a basis for their attribution of intention:

(27) She [teacher] had the table right beside her.

One subject 'placed' the hearer puppet alongside an activity when he reported

(28) Because the student was standing by the block table.

This subject had paraphrased the target utterance as a Question, 'do you want to play with the blocks?' rather than as a Request, thus rendering his reconstruction of the scenario's proxemics in a manner consistent with his apparent illocutionary interpretation of the stimulus utterance.

A very small number of responses to this interview item made reference to an illocutionary act or process, and mostly made simple reference to a speech act category, as in:

(29) By the questions she asks.

Finally, two responses made reference to pragmatic features of discourse. The first of these dealt with politeness conventions:

(30) Because the little girl probably doesn't like Art and the Art teacher is saying please because she wants her to.

The second involved an extended explanation of how pragmatic indirectness can be used to allow participants to save face:

(31) Well, it's hard to explain. She said it, but said it in words not saying it but she said it in her words. It's hard to explain. She said it in a different way than you usually say it but she wouldn't say it so it would insult the kid.

Discussion

The first aim of the present study was to describe the types of intentions younger school-aged children attributed to Speakers in conversational settings. We addressed this aim in two steps: first, by determining from the paraphrase task what illocutionary intent children imputed to the target utterances presented to them, and second, by asking in the interview why children thought the Speaker said what she did. Results of the paraphrase task showed that the majority of children understood the target utterances as one form or other of directive, in keeping with the design of the stimulus context, which was intended to predispose subjects to a directive uptake of the target utterance. Results of the probe question concerning Speaker's motivation revealed that children justified their attribution of illocutionary intent by mentioning a felicity condition for the imputed illocutionary act, together with mention of social role of speaker or hearer, or of an institutional routine. The question of whether the motivations mapped onto illocutionary acts mentioned in the paraphrase task was explored by cross-tabulation of the two sets of responses. A qualitative analysis of the main categories of motivation showed a good degree of fit between illocutionary act and speaker motivation obtained.

The second aim of the study was to investigate the extent to which children understood their own linguistic pragmatic comprehension processes. This we undertook by means of a further question in the clinical interview, asking children how they knew what they had said in response to the preceding probe question about speaker motivation. While a wide range of bases for the speaker intention justifications was offered, the largest category found was reference to the locution itself, mainly just the fact that the utterance had occurred, but also to the form of utterance. This is in line with findings of children's early sensitivity to the pragmatic implications of linguistic form (Bates, 1976; Becker, 1981; Ledbetter & Dent, 1988; Wilkinson *et al.*, 1984; Garton & Pratt, 1990). It also may lend support to one aspect of Baroni & Axia's (1989) finding that 7-year-olds were only beginning to move beyond attention to the linguistic form of an utterance to a conscious understanding of a pragmatic rule when they identified a speaker of a target utterance and justified their identifications. Nonetheless, a sufficiently-wide range of non-linguistic categories was employed by our sample to call into question recent findings (Abbeduto *et al.*, 1992; Bernicot & Laval, 1993) that children in the present age bracket show relatively poorly-developed ability to take participants' intentions into account. Moreover, evidence is emerging to show that the ability to consider conversational participants' intentions, attitutudes and face is socialized from a reasonably early age (Becker, 1988b; Becker, 1993).

The present results seem to run counter to those of Abbeduto *et al.*, 1992. However, despite the sophistication of design and procedure employed in that study, it may well have been that the failure of their younger subjects to respond correctly to the stimuli was an artifact of the cognitive and linguistic complexity of the task itself. First, it required a sophisticated semantic discrimination amongst Noun Phrases of varied definiteness ('NP number n' vs.'any of the NPs' vs. simply 'NPs'), as well as an application of that discrimination in pragmatic terms in order to formulate a response in keeping with the probable goal of the speaker. Abbeduto *et al.* allow the possibility that the 6–9-year-olds' difficulties lay in one or other of these domains. In addition, nonsense terms and items were used as the object of the exchange, a telephone conversation was required to answer the 'customer's' enquiry, and the child was required to enact the role of merchant, all three demands, when combined, adding computational complexity probably of an order beyond the general social experience (cf. Donaldson, 1978) and representational capability of many of the younger subjects. The researchers raise the important question of whether it will be possible to demonstrate younger age groups' ability to map speech act comprehension onto interpersonal goals in some simpler fashion, using more familiar settings or materials, and point to the inherent complexity in the actual use of awareness of participants' intentions in conversational settings.

It may be that the present study has succeeded in tapping children's recognition of, and ability to identify participant's goals and intentions, but not necessarily their ability to mobilize these understandings in complex and extended conversational interactions of the sorts devised by Abbeduto *et al.* and Bernicot & Laval. Clearly, further studies employing a sufficiently-wide range of methods (Clark, 1978), particularly are indicated. When settings and tasks are employed which are truly interesting and make intuitive sense to children (Donaldson, 1978), we may expect a more representative sample of children's abilities in the pragmatic and conversational domain. Further, the present study, along with the recent work cited, has allowed us to refine the broad question of whether younger school-aged children can take participant's goals and intentions into account. We are probably now in a position to ask at least three questions in this domain: we may investigate the *extent* to which participant intentions are employed (cf. Hickman *et al.*, 1993), the degree of complexity of representation of intentions and goals possible for children (cf. Baroni & Axia, 1989), and, finally, the contexts in which such performances can or cannot occur.

In conclusion, the present study found that regardless of illocutionary uptake to a particular utterance, the children seen appeared able to employ a good grasp of a speaker's intentional state when they were ascertaining illocutionary point of an utterance performed in context. These intentional states included speakers' attitudes, and goals, participants' roles, and institutional knowledge. Moreover, children reported employing a wide range of cues in order to attribute such intentional states to Speakers, including knowledge about both general and social cognition, social roles, proxemic and kinesic states, utterances and their form, illocutionary acts and their functions, interpretive processes, and pragmatic strategies including maintenance of politeness and face. Finally, children's justifications of a speaker's motivation in performing an utterance appeared consistent with their own illocutionary uptake, and were therefore principled in their basis.

References

Abbeduto, L., Nuccio Bibler, J., Al-Mabuk, R., Rotto, P. and Maas, F. (1992) Interpreting and responding to a spoken language: Children's recognition and use of a speaker's goal. *Journal of Child Language* 19, 677–93.

Baroni, M. R. and Axia, G. (1989) Children's meta-pragmatic abilities and the identification of polite and impolite requests. *First Language* 9, 285–97.

Bates, E. (1976) *Language and Context: The Acquisition of Pragmatics.* New York: Academic Press.

Becker, J. A. (1981) Preschoolers' judgments of speaker status based on requests. Paper presented at the Biennial Meeting of the Society for Research in Child Development, Boston.

— (1988a) I can't talk, I'm dead: Preschoolers' spontaneous metapragmatic comments. *Discourse Processes* 11, 457–67.

— (1988b) The success of parents' indirect techniques for teaching their preschoolers pragmatic skills. *First Language* 8, 173–82.

— (1993) Mothers' beliefs about the role of indirectness in teaching their preschoolers to say 'please'. Paper presented at the Sixth International Congress for the Study of Child Language, Trieste.

Bernicot, J. and Laval, V. (1993) Promises in children: Comprehension, metapragmatic knowledge and adaptation to the situation. Paper presented at the Sixth International Congress for the Study of Child Language, Trieste.

Clark, E. V. (1978) Awareness of language: Some evidence from what children say and do. In: A. Sinclair, R.J. Jarvella and J.M. Levelt (eds). *The Child's Conception of Language* Berlin: Springer-Verlag.

Donaldson, M. (1978) *Children's Minds.* Glasgow: Fontana/Collins.

Garton, A. F. and Pratt, C. (1990) Children's pragmatic judgements of direct and indirect requests. *First Language* 10, 51–9.

Grice, H. P. (1975) Logic and conversation. In P. Cole & J. L. Morgan (eds), *Speech Acts: Syntax and Semantics*, Vol 3. New York: Academic Press.

Halliday, M.A.K. (1975) *Learning How to Mean.* London: Edward Arnold.

Hickman, M., Champaud, C. and Bassano, D. (1993) Pragmatics and metapragmatics in the development of epistemic modality: Evidence from French children' s reports of *think*-statements. *First Language* 13, 359–89.

James, S. (1975) Effect of listener age and situation on the politeness of children's directives. *Journal of Psycholinguistic Research* 7, 307–17.

Ledbetter, P. J. and Dent, C. H. (1988) Young children's sensitivity to direct and indirect requests' structures. *First Language* 8, 227–45.

Leonard, L. B. and Reid, L. (1979) Children's judgments of utterance appropriateness. *Journal of Speech and Hearing Research* 22, 500–15.

Levinson, S. C. (1983) *Pragmatics.* Cambridge: Cambridge University Press.

Reeder, K. (1983) Classifications of children's speech acts: A consumer's guide. *Journal of Pragmatics* 7, 679–94.

Reeder, K. and Wakefield, P. J. (1987) The development of young children's speech act comprehension: How much language is necessary? *Applied Psycholinguistics*, 8, 1–18.

Searle, J. R. (1969) *Speech Acts: An Essay in the Philosophy of Language.* Cambridge: Cambridge University Press.

— (1979) *Expression and Meaning.* Cambridge: Cambridge University Press.

Shatz, M. (1978) On the development of communicative understandings: An early strategy for interpreting and responding to messages. *Cognitive Psychology* 10, 271–301.

Shatz, M. and Gelman, R. (1973) The development of communication skills: Modifications in the speech of young children as a function of listener. *Monographs of the Society for Research in Child Development* 38 (5), serial no. 152.

Wilkinson, L. C., Wilkinson, A. C., Spinelli, F. and Chiang, C. P. (1984) Metalinguistic knowledge of pragmatic rules in school-age children. *Child Development* 55, 2130–140.

13 The Effectiveness of Therapy for Child Phonological Disorder: The Metaphon Approach

JENNIFER REID, MORAG L. DONALDSON, JANET HOWELL, ELIZABETH C. DEAN AND ROBERT GRIEVE

Phonological Disorder

Children who have a phonological disorder have problems with the production (and possibly also the perception) of speech sound contrasts, which results in their speech having poor intelligibility, even though it is usually fairly fluent. This disorder is amongst the most common forms of specific language impairment, especially in the preschool and early school years (and it can also occur in children whose language difficulties are associated with other problems, such as a general developmental delay). Although there is evidence that pure phonological disorder is more likely to resolve spontaneously than other forms of specific language impairment (Bishop & Edmundson, 1987), there is also evidence to suggest that children with phonological disorders may be at increased risk of experiencing reading problems (Silva, Williams & McGee, 1987). Furthermore, research emphasising the role of phonological awareness in the development of reading skills (Bradley & Bryant, 1983) implies that children with phonological disorder may be at a disadvantage in learning to read. For these reasons, it is important to investigate how speech and language therapists could intervene effectively to resolve children's phonological disorders.

Traditional 'articulation therapy' approaches to the treatment of phonological disorder have tended to focus on improving children's perception and/or articulatory production within an essentially behavioural framework. More recently, however, there has been a shift towards therapeutic approaches which place greater emphasis on the child's phonological system and therefore on higher level cognitive processes. For example, Grunwell (1983: 167) argues that: '. . . Changes in speech production need to take place, not so much in the mouth, but in the mind of the child. The aim of treatment is to effect cognitive re-organisation rather than articulatory re-training . . .' An underlying assumption of such approaches is that children's speech errors are systematic, and one way of characterising this systematicity is in terms of phonological processes which apply to classes of speech sounds rather to individual phonetic segments. For instance, one child may have a phonological process involving fronting of velars (such that *cup* is pronounced as [tʌp] and *big* as [bɪd]), and another child may have a phonological process involving stopping of fricatives (such that *fish* is pronounced as [pɪt] and *kiss* as [kɪt]). The goal of therapy is to help the child to change these phonological processes towards the phonological rules which underpin adults' speech. Hewlett (1990) postulates several requirements which have to be met in order for phonological rule revision to occur. These include the child having (a) awareness of the insufficiency of the current production, (b) a desire to change the current production and (c) knowledge of the relevant crucial articulatory targets. Metaphon therapy aims to help children meet these three requirements.

Metaphon Therapy

The basic premise of Metaphon therapy is that phonological change can be brought about by utilising and enhancing phonological and communicative awareness. To assist in this process, Metaphon therapy provides activities which help the children to realise that words are composed of individual sounds and that these sounds have certain properties which enable them to be distinguished from and grouped with other sounds. The children are then given the opportunity to use this knowledge in activities designed to show them that they can increase the listener's understanding of what they say by making corrections, in other words by using repair strategies.

It is an essential feature of Metaphon that the provision of relevant linguistic knowledge takes place in a therapeutic environment which maximises the child's learning opportunities. In essence Metaphon subscribes to the view that children learn through active problem solving. This influences the type of therapeutic activities that are used in this therapy, the way these activities are presented to the children, and the interactional patterns between child and therapist. The therapist provides learning opportunities and facilitates the child's reflection on the speech sound system through conversation, communicative activities and graded feedback. A detailed description of the theoretical basis of Metaphon can be found in Howell and Dean (1991).

Practical application of Metaphon consists of two closely interrelated phases. In Phase 1 the children's attention is drawn to those contrastive features of the speech sound system which are relevant to the particular simplifying process which is to be targeted. A first step in this process is to introduce the child to terms which describe the salient phonetic features which are to be the focus of attention, using vocabulary which is meaningful to the child. If we take stopping of fricatives as an example, the words 'long' and 'short' may be used to refer to fricatives and stops. Therapy starts with games which illustrate the contrast between the two concepts, such as pinning long and short bananas on a tree. This will be followed by activities which focus on the contrast in non-speech sounds, such as making long and short blasts on a trumpet. The next stage is for child and therapist to take it in turns to be speaker and listener, producing and responding to a range of stops and fricatives. The speaker produces any stop or fricative and the listener carries out a corresponding activity, such as drawing long or short stems on flowers. At the end of Phase 1, minimal pair words (e.g. *sew/toe*), produced by the therapist, are used to facilitate the child's awareness of sounds in words, and to show the child that changes in phonetic features correspond to changes in meaning.

Phase 2 of Metaphon aims to encourage children to transfer what they have learned in Phase 1 to communicative situations and to develop their communicative awareness. Opportunities are provided for the children to monitor their own speech, and to make any self corrections that are required. Child and therapist once again take it in turns to be speaker and listener. A picturable minimal pair is selected, for example *tea/sea*, six to eight copies of each picture are placed face down in a pile and one pair is placed face up on the table. The speaker selects a picture from the pile and names it and the listener chooses from the two pictures on the table according to the word *he/she* has heard. The minimal pair words are usually referred to as 'secret messages', an enticing term for the children. Once the child becomes proficient at making distinctions between minimal pairs, the words are put into a constant sentence context. For instance, the speaker may give the listener instructions to 'hide the *tea/sea*'.

Initial Metaphon Efficacy Study

This study (Howell, Hill, Dean & Waters, 1993) employed a multiple-baseline, single case study design repeated across 13 children with phonological disorder. Each child acted as his or her own control in that two of the child's simplifying processes were targeted in therapy while a third process was left untreated to serve as a control measure. The children's ages ranged from 3;7 to 4;7 (mean age 4;1) and they were all treated by the same speech and language therapist.

The results from this study were broadly encouraging. On assessments of phonological production and phonological awareness, the children's post-therapy scores were significantly higher than their pre-therapy scores. Also, the targeted processes showed declines which were clearly related in time to the onset of therapy. However, individual children showed different patterns of change, with some showing change only in the targeted processes and others showing change in the control process as well.

These findings, although promising, leave several important questions unanswered:

(1) How should changes in the control process be interpreted? These could indicate either that the children were generalising their learning from the targeted processes to the control process (in which case Metaphon could be regarded as particularly powerful), or that the changes in the targeted processes were not really brought about by the therapy since the control processes also changed (in which case Metaphon could be regarded as ineffective).

(2) How might the individual differences in responses to Metaphon be explained?

(3) Does the effectiveness of Metaphon generalise to a larger sample of children and therapists?

These questions cannot be answered on the basis of evidence from single case studies. In order to complement and extend the case study findings it was therefore considered necessary to conduct a more extensive study with a larger sample of children and therapists and a treated/untreated group design. As well as addressing the three questions outlined above, the group study aims to investigate a further question:

(4) Are both phases of Metaphon required in order to bring about phonological change?

Current Study: Design and Method

This large-scale ongoing study is funded by the Medical Research Council. Therapy is being delivered by 20 speech and language therapists who have been trained to use the Metaphon approach and who work in a variety of National Health Service clinics in 6 different regions of Britain. Approximately 100 pre-school children with phonological disorder are participating: in this paper, we report on some of the results from 30 of these children. Subjects are selected according to the following criteria:

• no previous speech therapy

• aged 3;6–5;6 years at time of pre-therapy assessment

- monolingual English-speaking background

- normal hearing at the time of the study

- no known cognitive, neurological or anatomical impairments

- standard score above −1.0 on RDLS Verbal Comprehension Scale (Reynell, 1985)

- standard score of 85 or less on the Edinburgh Articulation Test (Anthony, Bogle, Ingram & McIsaac, 1971)

The study uses primarily a between-subjects, group design, in order to allow comparisons of change in treated and untreated groups. However, some elements of a case study design have been retained: within subjects, we carry out pre- and post-treatment measures of not only the phonological process which has been targeted for treatment but also another 'control' process. The design also incorporates a variety of individual difference measures in order to investigate their contribution to differences in outcome and allow analysis of covariance.

Subjects are randomly allocated to one of four conditions:

Group 1:   treatment condition: 6 sessions phase 1 Metaphon

Group 2:   treatment condition: 10 sessions phases 1 and 2 Metaphon

Group 3:   control condition: 6 weeks no treatment

Group 4:   control condition: 10 weeks no treatment

Children in the first experimental condition receive 6 sessions of Metaphon therapy, phase 1 only, that is, activities relating only to establishment of a shared vocabulary, categorisation of non-speech and speech sounds and detection and classification of sounds-in-words. In the second experimental group, the children receive 10 sessions of Metaphon therapy, and these include phase 2 activities, that is, the use of minimal pairs in a communicative framework with the emphasis on communicative effectiveness. In both experimental groups, the children attend for 30 minute sessions once a week, and only one simplifying process is targeted. Experimental group 1, therefore, receives a total of 3 hours of therapy, whereas group 2 receives 5 hours in total. A battery of assessments is carried out before therapy commences and re-assessments follow immediately after the therapy period.

The children in the third group act as untreated controls for the 6-session treatment group. They are assessed then re-assessed after 6 weeks without intervention. Similarly, the fourth group are re-assessed after 10 weeks without therapy and act as untreated controls for the 10-session treatment group.

The assessment battery comprises a range of measures which fall into three categories:

a) *Dependent Measures* which intervention is expected to affect. These were assessed before and immediately after the treatment/no treatment period for all groups. Two tests were selected as measures of phonological production: the Edinburgh Articulation Test (EAT) (Anthony *et al.*, 1971) and a phonological process analysis from the Metaphon Resource Pack (Dean, Howell, Hill & Waters, 1990). A further two tests were devised to measure awareness of onset and rhyme, both aspects of phonological awareness (Reid, Grieve, Dean, Donaldson & Howell, 1993).

b) *Control Measures* which intervention is not expected to affect. These consisted of a word order awareness task (Reid *et al.*, 1993), as a measure of non-phonological, linguistic awareness, and the British Picture Vocabulary Scales (Dunn, Dunn, Whetton & Pintillie, 1982), as a linguistic measure which correlates strongly with verbal intelligence. These were also assessed before and immediately after the treatment/no treatment period for all groups.

c) *Other Variables and Factors* which may influence outcome. These were assessed once only, before the treatment/no treatment period, for all groups, and comprised the Reynell Developmental Language Scales (Reynell, 1985) and tests of auditory discrimination, motor speech production ability and 'cognitive style'. Other factors include sex, age, social class, therapist and geographical location.

The individual difference measures will eventually be used to explore possible reasons for different patterns of response to Metaphon therapy, but for the purposes of this chapter, we shall focus on group differences and in particular, on the following hypotheses:

(1) If Metaphon is effective, children in the 6-session treatment and/or the 10-session treatment group will show more improvement than children in the control groups in phonological production (as measured by phonological process analysis and/or EAT).

(2) If both phases of Metaphon are required for the treatment to be effective, only children in the 10-session treatment group will show more improvement than children in the control groups.

(3) If Metaphon brings about change by harnessing and enhancing phonological awareness, the experimental groups will show more improvement than the control groups between pre- and post-test scores on the metaphonological tasks.

(4) If Metaphon is specific in its effect, the differences between pre- and post-test scores on the control measures (word order awareness; receptive vocabulary) will be no greater in the experimental groups than in the control groups.

Current Study: Results and Discussion

As data are still being collected and coded, and we do not yet have equal or balanced numbers of subjects in all four groups, the results reported below are based on a subset of 30 subjects, in which both experimental and control subjects from the same therapist were available. As the resulting sample sizes are small, and variance in scores on some tests is clearly unequal across groups, we attempt to draw only tentative conclusions, based on initial data exploration and non-parametric tests.

Do any of the groups show significant increases in phonological production?

If we look first for change in scores on the EAT, we see a significant increase in standard scores only in the group which received 10 sessions, and both phases of Metaphon (see Table 13.1). Of course, the fact that this group showed improvement whereas the 6 session treatment group did not could be due either to the effect of phase 2 Metaphon or simply to the longer treatment period.

Table 13.1 Median EAT standard scores

Group	N	Score pre-	Score post-	Significance level of T
6 sessions therapy, phase 1	8	74	72	*n.s.*
6 weeks no therapy	8	80	75	*n.s.*
10 seesions therapy, phase 1& 2	7	75	84	*p=0.02*
10 weeks no therapy	7	80	87	*n.s.*

However, when we look at changes in *raw* scores on the same test (see Table 13.2), we see that the median scores for all the groups, with the exception of the 6 week control group, increase from pre- to post-assessments, and that these differences are significant (Wilcoxon signed ranks test). This pattern, with significant changes in the 10 week control group as well as in the treatment groups, suggests strongly that at least *some* of the observed changes are maturational. Even over a period of time as short as 10 weeks, children's productions are not static, but continue to move towards the adult target system.

There is a very marked degree of individual variation in EAT results. Within each group, including control groups, there are at least one or two children who make quite dramatic progress between pre- and post-testing. There are also individuals who make no progress at all, and whose standardised scores deteriorate as a consequence .

Table 13.2 Median EAT raw scores

Group	N	Score pre-	Score post-	Significance level of T
6 sessions therapy, phase 1	8	24	30	*p*=0.02
6 weeks no therapy	8	28	28	*n.s.*
10 seesions therapy, phase 1& 2	7	26	34	*p*=0.02
10 weeks no therapy	7	27	39	*p*=0.01

Turning now to the other measure of phonological production, that is the number of times a phonological process occurred in the sample of words elicited using the relevant Metaphon Resource Pack 'probe', more evidence of ongoing maturation emerges.

Table 13.3 Median percentage occurrence of phonological process A (the process targeted in therapy for children in the treated groups)

Group	N	Score pre-	Score post-	Significance level of T
6 sessions therapy, phase 1	8	76	87	*n.s.*
6 weeks no therapy	8	82	80	*p*=0.04
10 seesions therapy, phase 1& 2	7	100	63	*p*=0.04
10 weeks no therapy	7	89	71	*p*=0.02

Significant decreases in percentage occurrence of process A (the process targeted in therapy for children in the treated groups) occur in control groups as well as the 10 session treatment group (see Table 13.3).

The somewhat lower pre-test score of the 6 session treatment group is a little misleading and requires some explanation. While the group includes 3 children with scores at or near 100%, it also includes children in whom more than one process is operating in the same environment, such as a child who either fronts or stops palato-alveolars, or another who either deletes or fronts velars. As the percentage score for these subjects is based on the occurrence of only *one* of these processes (i.e. the process selected for therapy), the pre-test scores of this group are artificially low, since their productions of the target sounds are not 'correct' on any occasion. The apparent *increase* in the post-test occurrence is due to more systematic use of one process and decline in use of the other process. For example, the child who either fronts or stops palato-alveolars may show a decrease in use of stopping (the more immature process) and a consequent increase in use of fronting (the targeted process). Such changes are likely to be maturational in origin rather than due to intervention.

That the minimal change in the median scores in the 6 week control group reaches significance may appear perplexing at first sight. Of course, the Wilcoxon test is not a test of differences in the median, but rather takes into account the direction of changes between the two sets of scores. Closer inspection of individual scores reveals that one child showed an increase, two children made no change and the remaining five children showed decreases. Of these five, two children made dramatic improvements. One child appeared to eradicate word-initial stopping of fricatives, while in the second, fronting of velars in all word positions reduced from 85% to 11% .

In contrast to the previous finding, changes in the 'control' process do not reach significance in any of the groups (see Table 13.4). Why should this process show less evidence of change than process A, even in the untreated groups? In order to ensure that the research was conducted in a clinical situation that was as close to 'the real world' as possible, therapists were encouraged to exercise their own clinical judgement in selecting processes, that is, using criteria such as contribution to unintelligibility, degree of immaturity/atypicality, variability and whether the child is able to produce sounds in isolation. In practice, process A, the one selected for therapy in the treated groups, tends to be the one which is either the most devastating to intelligibility or the most developmentally immature. In the control groups, process A was the process which the therapist would go on to target after administration of the post-tests. Thus, for most children, process B will end up being of a rather different developmental status to process A. These early analyses have convinced us of the need to use something other than percentage occurrence of an untreated process as a measure of the extent to which change has generalised beyond the specific targets of intervention. Therefore, we are experimenting with quantification of the results of the Metaphon Resource Pack screening procedure as an alternative measure.

Table 13.4 Median percentage occurrence of phonological process B ('control' process, not selected for therapy)

Group	N	Score pre-	Score post-	Significance level of T
6 sessions therapy, phase 1	8	95	88	n.s.
6 weeks no therapy	8	97	83	n.s.
10 seesions therapy, phase 1& 2	7	85	63	n.s.
10 weeks no therapy	7	94	90	n.s.

Is there any evidence for the hypothesis that Metaphon therapy works by harnessing and developing children's knowledge and awareness of language, in particular, their phonological awareness?

Only in the 10 session treatment group are there any significant changes between pre- and post-test scores on the metalinguistic assessments. Results for this group are given in Table 13.5.

Table 13.5 Median scores on selected tests (10 session treatment group)

Test	Pre-therapy score	Post-therapy score	Significance level of T
phoneme awareness	0.42	0.58	$p=0.03$
rhyme awareness	0.75	0.70	n.s.
word order awareness	0.80	0.80	n.s.
BPVS (raw score)	33	35	n.s.

As well as the apparently specific nature of the change in metalinguistic ability, this change occurs in the context of no significant change in vocabulary score, not even in the raw scores, which might be expected to show maturational changes over this period. Only phoneme awareness appears to have increased to a significant degree, and this only in the group receiving 'the full course' of treatment. This is some preliminary evidence in support of the hypothesis that Metaphon is tapping specific aspects of phonological awareness.

Conclusions

The finding that significant amounts of maturational change occur over a 10 week period, casts serious doubt on the results of single case study designs, in which *any* change in phonological production observed during and/or after a period of intervention is taken to be an intervention effect. Furthermore, the high degree of individual variation already evident, even in this subset of the final sample, demonstrates the value of controlled group studies of this kind.

There is some preliminary evidence of accelerated phonological development in children receiving 'the full course' of Metaphon therapy over 10 sessions, and changes in phonological production appear to be accompanied by an increase in metaphonological ability, as measured by a task which is related to, but nevertheless different from any of the Metaphon therapy activities. It is also evident, though, that there is considerable individual variation in patterns of phonological change, both in treated and in control groups. Subsequent analyses on the completed data set will aim to explicate these patterns and their implications for theory and practice.

References

Anthony, A. and Bogle, D., *et al.* (1971) *Edinburgh Articulation Test.* Edinburgh: Livingstone.

Bishop, D. and Edmundson, A. (1987) Language-impaired 4-year-olds: distinguishing transient from persistent impairment. *Journal of Speech and Hearing Disorders* 52: 156–73.

Bradley, L. and Bryant, P.E. (1983) Categorising sounds and learning to read: a causal connection. *Nature* 301: 419–21.

Dean, E. C., Howell, J. *et al.* (1990) *Metaphon Resource Pack.* Windsor: NFER-Nelson.

Dunn, L. M., Dunn, L. *et al.* (1982) *British Picture Vocabulary Scale.* Windsor: NFER-Nelson.

Grunwell, P. (1983) *Phonological Therapy: Premises, Principles and Procedures.* XIX Congress of IALP, Edinburgh, University of Edinburgh.

Hewlett, N. (1990) Processes of development and production. In P. Grunwell (ed.) *Developmental Speech Disorders.* Edinburgh: Churchill Livingstone.

Howell, J. and Dean, E.C. (1991) *Treating Phonological Disorders in Children: Metaphon-Theory to Practice.* London: Whurr.

Howell, J., Hill, A. *et al.* (1993) Increasing metalinguistic awareness to assist phonological change. In D.J. Messer & G.J. Turner (eds.) *Critical Influences on Child Language Acquisition and Development.* London: Macmillan.

Reid, J., Grieve, R., Dean, E.C., Donaldson, M.L. and Howell, J. (1993) Linguistic awareness in young children. In J. Clibbens & B. Pendleton (eds.) *Proceedings of the Child Language Seminar 1993.* Plymouth: University of Plymouth.

Reynell, J. (1985) *Reynell Language Development Scales.* Windsor, Berks.: NFER-Nelson.

Silva, P. A., Williams, S. *et al.* (1987) A longitudinal study of children with developmental language delay at age three: later intelligence, reading and behaviour problems. *Developmental Medicine and Child Neurology* 29, 630–40.

14 Functional Category Cueing[1]

MILTON TAYLOR

Introduction: The Functional Parameterisation Hypothesis

This chapter is an attempt to bring together two apparently very different models in order to explain the crosslinguistic and cross-categorial development of Functional Categories (FCs).

According to the *Functional Parametrisation Hypothesis* (Chomsky, 1991: 419, following Borer, 1984; Fukui, 1988), all parameterisation is restricted to the lexical properties of FCs. Three types of FC parameters have been posited: *c-selection, feature,* and *presence/absence* parameters. The c-selection properties of each FC in a particular language determine the ordering of projections in clauses. For example, Ouhalla (1991) argues that in Berber, Tense c-selects Agreement, whereas Agreement c-selects Tense in Chichewa, affecting the ordering of elements in the languages:

(1a) ad-   y-   segh Mohand ijn teddart

     will(T)-3ms(Agr)-buy Mohand one house

     'Mohand will buy a house'   (Berber: Ouhalla, 1991: 57)

(1b) mtsuko- u-   na-   gw -a

     waterpot-SP(Agr)-Past(T)-fall-ASP

     'The waterpot fell'   (Chichewa: Baker, 1988)

Ouhalla (1991: 77) also argues that FCs may vary in terms of their features. For example, in Welsh, Aspect is nominal, so Aspect and (inherently verbal) Tense morphemes may not attach to the same stem; however Aspect is verbal in Kinyarwanda, so Tense and Aspect morphemes may appear on the same stem:

(2a) roedd   Adrian yn   mynd i'r parti gwyllt

      be-past(T) Adrian ASP go to the party wild

      'Adrian was going to the wild party'   (Welsh)

(2b) umwaana y- a-   taa-   ye igitabo mu maazi

      child SP-Past(T)-throw-ASP book   in water

      'The child has thrown the book into the water'

                                        (Kinyarwanda: Baker, 1988)

Far from being required in all languages and all structures by UG, the presence or absence of FCs is also open to parametric variation. For example, Subject Agreement is purported to be absent in languages such as Japanese (Fukui, 1986), Chinese (Aoun, 1986) and Kikongo (Radford, 1990). It is purported to be absent in English infinitival clauses, but present in European Portuguese infinitival clauses (Madeira, 1993). Tense is purported to be absent from Inuktitut verbal structures (Fortesque, 1984: 272; Shaer, 1989), and absent from nominals and gerundival clauses in most languages (Ouhalla, 1991), but present in Japanese nominals (Fukuda & Fukuda, 1994). The presence of FCs varies from language to language, and from structure to structure within languages.

The Development of Functional Categories

There has been much debate in recent years about the presence or otherwise of FCs at the initial state, and during the early multiword stages. The appearance of FCs in spontaneous speech varies crosslinguistically, and FCs do not appear to be mastered all at the same time within one language. For example, Tense and/or Agreement inflections are argued to be mastered before 2;0 in Japanese, French, Turkish and Italian (e.g. Clancy, 1985: 425; Weissenborn, 1988; Aksu-Koc & Slobin, 1985; Pizzuto & Caselli, 1992), but not in English, Polish, Swedish, German, Greek, Spanish or Welsh (Radford, 1990; Smoczynska, 1985: 617; Platzack, 1990; Clahsen, 1991; Tsimpli, 1991; Pina, 1984; Aldridge *et al.*, 1994). Within languages, it has been argued that Aspect appears before Tense, which appears before Subject Agreement, which appears before Complementiser in English (Radford, 1987; Radford & Aldridge, 1987; Tsimpli, 1992). This is expected if we assume that FCs have c-selection parameters, and that FCs cannot select another FC which the child has not yet acquired, which predicts that a FC will never be fully acquired unless its complements have been acquired. Therefore, 'higher' dominating FCs will always be acquired later than 'lower' daughter FCs.

However, the *crosslinguistic* variation in the onset of FCs cannot be explained by their hierarchical positions in particular structures. Moreover, there is considerable crosslinguistic evidence of an 'optional infinitive' stage when children are beginning to demonstrate knowledge of FCs (Wexler, 1993). Briefly, children will move finite verbs appropriately and produce nonfinite verbs in base postions, demonstrating their knowledge that Tense/Agreement inflections stand for Tense/Agreement FCs, and that the features of these categories must be checked at s-structure. However, they do not produce finite verbs in all matrix clauses: finite verbs seem to be produced optionally. We might infer from this that Tense/Agreement projections are generated optionally at this stage, or that these FCs are present, but their feature parameters have not been fully set to [+STRONG] (Wexler, 1993). Children are wavering between the settings (3a) and (3b):

(3)   In matrix declarative clauses, Subject Agreement has:

(a) weak features (no verb movement)

(b) strong features (verb movement)

This is a problem for traditional 'all-or-none' parameter-setting theories, which do not predict the lengthy and protracted period it takes children to converge to setting (3b) in those languages that require it. The child should not bounce from (3a) to (3b) to (3a) to (3b). But in the optional infinitive stage, this is precisely what happens. There is no sudden jump from (3a) to (3b); instead, there is a lot of bungee-jumping going on.

A possible answer to this problem is that the gradual increase in the production of (moved) finite matrix verbs is a function of affix learning and not parameter setting (Taylor, 1995a). Under the *Affix Learning* hypothesis of the optional infinitive stage, the feature parameter setting (3b) has already been set, and optionality of inflected verbs is a function or affix learning. So the optional infinitive stage is subsumed to the domain of affix learning, which is a lexical matter and not a parametrical matter, as argued by most parameter-setting theorists. However, one might argue, following Pizzuto & Caselli, (1992; 1993), that parameter setting is *explanatorily redundant* in describing the optional infinitive stage, if this is the case.

In summary, we have two outstanding questions: why does the onset and rate or FC development vary from language to language, and can we account for the initial optionality of FC surface features (grammatical morphemes) in a model of parameter setting? In the next two sections I shall describe two different models which answer each question; in the final section, I shall show how they may be brought together into one model.

The Competition Model: The Rate and Onset of FC Development

Researchers have recently begun to take more notice of the role of language processing in language acquisition. The idea makes sense: all the time the child is being exposed to input, she is trying to understand what she hears and make herself understood to adults — not just setting parameters. One framework which attempts to model both language processing and language acquisition is the *Competition Model* (CM) (e.g. MacWhinney & Bates, 1989). One assumption of the CM is that people use cues to process what they hear. Cues can come from any level of linguistic structure (phonology, semantics, morphology, word order) and the utterance context. These cues are processed simultaneously and may interact with each other, converging if they lead to identical interpretations, and competing if they lead to conflicting interpretations. If there is competition between cues, those cues which are generally most *available* (present, frequent, phonetically salient) and/or most *reliable* (leading to a consistent interpretation, always present for that interpretation) will win out over cues which are less available and/or reliable. *Cue Strength* is a product of a cue's availability multiplied by reliability (McDonald, 1989; MacWhinney, 1989: 94), and as such may be measured probablistically.

Crosslinguistic studies of adult sentence processing have shown that the relative usefulness of grammatical morphemes as processing cues varies from language to language (see Hernandez *et al.*, 1994 for a review). For example, English speakers presented with (4a) show a tendency to choose the first argument as the agent of the sentence, despite the conflicting Agreement features on the auxiliary: the order of arguments is a more important cue to agenthood than morphological cues. Italian speakers, on the other hand, when presented with (4b), show a tendency to assign agenthood to the second argument, paying more attention to the verb inflection than to the argument order (Bates *et al.*, 1984):

(4a) The eraser are chasing the boys

(4b) La gomma cocciano i ragazzi

　　　the eraser   chase-3pl the boys

Verb agreement morphology seems to be a stronger cue than argument order to agenthood in Italian; the opposite is true for English. Italian has a rich and salient verbal agreement paradigm, unlike English: Agreement morphology has more cue availability in Italian than in English.

The CM predicts that children, like adults, attempt to utilise and use cues with the highest strength when they are processing input on-line. It might be additionally stipulated that, due to less competent processing, children place a heavier reliance on high-strength cues to the expense of cues which are lower in strength, compared to adults. It certainly follows that, where the surface realisations of FCs are *higher* in cue strength, they will be acquired earlier and faster than where the surface realisations of FCs are *lower* in cue strength. This predicts both crosslinguistic and cross-category variation in development. Grammatical morphology differs in cue strength from language to language, and different grammatical morphemes within the same language differ in their relative cue strengths. It might be predicted that languages with richer, phonetically salient paradigms for agreement morphemes facilitate the acquisition of the FC Agreement more than languages with sparse, unsalient agreement morphology. Indeed, grammatical morphemes appear and are mastered much earlier in Italian than they are in English (Guasti, 1993; Hyams, 1984; Pizzuto & Caselli, 1992).

Also, it might be predicted that FC realisations which have higher cue strength will develop earlier and quicker than FC realisations which have lower cue strength. Negation in English, which may be expressed as an emphatic stressed 'not', or as a clitic on a modal/auxiliary triggering a salient vowel change, or as a syllabic clitic, or in salient initial positions (5a-d), has higher cue availability than past tense {-ed}, which is often nonsyllabic and hardly ever stressed; past time may be inferred by the context if the {-ed} affix is not perceived (Taylor, 1995b):

(5a) I'm not responding to that

(5b) I shall/shan't rewrite my thesis

(5c) We would/wouldn't dream of it

(5d) Not that you're going to like this, but...

(6)   We were supposed to leave at half past nine, but we had had a
      'hunt the slipper' party the night before, and all morning
      mother was pacing up and down the park getting cross while we
      look for our shoes. We eventually found them in the microwave.

Even if the absence of an {-ed} is detected by a hearer of (6), she will detect an ungrammaticality rather than interpret the action as taking place in non-past time. Here, a contextual cue overrides a morphological cue. It is hard to imagine contextual cues overriding the negator 'not' in the same way as this; this is because 'not' is extremely high in cue strength. It follows from this that {-ed} is a much weaker processing cue than 'not', and that 'not' should appear earlier, and be mastered before, {-ed}; the FC NegP will be acquired earlier than the FC Tense in English, and negators should appear earlier and develop faster than {-ed}, modals and auxiliaries (as argued by Klima & Bellugi, 1966; Radford, 1990; Tsimpli, 1992).

The Genetic Algorithm Model and Functional Category Cueing

Assuming that the CM accounts for the crosslinguistic and cross-categorial variation in the acquisition of grammatical morphemes, is there anything which parameter-setting theories might have to say about this process? In this section, I shall briefly illustrate a model in which parameter values compete with each other for activation, the *Genetic Algorithm Model* (GA). The very name 'genetic algorithm' presupposes some element of competition and selection, and it is precisely these notions which the model exploits. It assumes that grammars are represented as 'parameter strings' of binary values (Clark, 1990; 1992; Clark & Roberts, 1993), as in (7), which shows two strings of eight parameters with exactly opposing values:

(7a) 0 0 1 1 0 1 0 1

(7b) 1 1 0 0 1 0 1 0

We might assume, for example, that the value of the presence parameter for Subject Agreement is set at 0 (absent) in English infinitival clauses, and set at 1 (present) in European Portuguese infinitival clauses. The GA model assumes that initially, *both* 0 and 1 settings of *all* parameters are available to the child, in competing parameter strings. The GA converges upon the target grammar by promoting those parameter strings which parse the input with fewest violations of UG principles (e.g. X-bar theory, the ECP), and penalising parameter strings which parse the input with more violations of these principles. 'Unfit' parameter strings are gradually weeded out until the child is left with a single string of parameter settings which parse the input with the minimum amount of violations.

Ability to parse the input with minimum UG violations is not the only thing which the GA takes into account when assigning fitness: *constants* penalise superset grammars and grammars which require longer movement chains, following the Subset and Economy principles (Berwick, 1985; Wexler & Manzini, 1987; Chomsky, 1993; Collins, 1994). The *Subset Constant* prevents strings which generate superset grammars from getting a high weighting too quickly, even if they parse the input successfully. Gibson & Wexler (1994) argue that if a child acquiring a non-V2 language assumes she is acquiring a V2 language, her grammar will fall into *local maxima*, a superset state which cannot be reversed by positive evidence. Clark & Roberts (1993: 324) predict that the GA initially penalises V2 parameter-strings, and hence children acquiring V2 languages will go through a stage in which they do not move verbs into C (e.g. as observed by Clahsen, 1991), giving a non-target (i.e. non-V2) grammar a preferential setting.

As far as Economy is concerned, the GA would give the feature parameter value [+Agr-weak] a higher weighting than the opposing value [+Agr-strong] because the former value does not force verb movement at s-structure, whereas the latter one does (see 3), and is thus more economical. The less economical value will win out during acquisition if there is evidence for Subject Agreement in the target language. Winning out is a protracted process, during which the two settings of this parameter compete with each other for activation. So the bungee-jump behaviour seen in the optional infinitive stage is not only explained, but *predicted* by the GA model. Children would know the difference between finite and nonfinite verbs and place them in correct positions, moving verbs whenever [+Agr-strong] is activated during the production process, and not when [+Agr-weak] is activated. Bungee-jumping continues until [+Agr-strong] has won out over [+Agr-weak], getting less and less frequent as development progresses.

The GA model, therefore, offers a theory of parameter-setting which does explain optional verb movement in child language, and which is a plausible alternative to the affix-learning hypothesis. But this doesn't mean that it is sufficient to explain crosslinguistic and cross-category variation in the acquisition of FCs. Indeed, Clark (1992: 132) argues that the child must be able to detect the effects of a parameter value in the input with sufficient frequency, in order to focus upon this parameter value. This is exactly the sort of appeal to phonetic availability and interpretative reliability which the Competition Model is making. Simply put, the cue strength of surface elements which express the properties of FC parameters determine the ease of acquisition of these parameters. I call this process *Functional Category Cueing*.

Functional Category Cueing: Number in Italian

Functional Category Cueing takes the notion of cue strength from the CM and constrains the CM with principles and parameters theory, using the genetic algorithm model. This process takes into account the evidence for an innate language acquisition device, the principles of UG, and the Subset and Economy constraints on parameter-setting. It also takes into account crosslinguistic and cross-category differences in the onset and rate of FC development; the influence of processing constraints, and predicts initial optionality or bungee-jump behaviour with verb movement. In this section we shall see how the model accounts for some data from Italian.

Although Agreement affixes appear in Italian well before age 2;0, studies have found a generally protracted development of *plural* forms relative to *singular* verbal agreement forms. In an elicited production task, Caselli *et al.*, (1993: 384) found that children aged 2;6 were significantly worse at producing plural than singular inflections in obligatory contexts (80% and 92% respectively). In a comprehension picture pointing task with 50% chance levels, the same group scored 75% for plurals and 93% for singulars — both above chance, but again a significant difference. Leonard *et al.*, (1992) studied a similar age group as language-matched controls for a group of language-impaired (LI) children, and found almost identical percentages, with the same patterns. The LI children, aged from

4 to 8 years, showed a marked difference between singulars and plurals: 93% and 50% respectively for production, 84%, 65% for comprehension. The most common error reported both in these studies and in spontaneous speech studies (Leonard *et al.*, 1987; Pizzuto & Caselli, 1992) is substitution of singular forms for plural forms, i.e. correct Tense, Gender, Person, but wrong Number.

Ritter (1993) argues that Number is an autonomous FC projection in some languages, and a feature of Agreement in others. If Number is a FC in Italian, we need to explain the protracted growth of a parameter value stating that Number is present. Since Number inflections always appear after Gender/Person inflections in Italian (8), we might infer (following Ouhalla, 1991) that Number is 'higher' in the clause hierarchy (9):

(8) *Verbs ending in:*   -are   -ere   -ire

                singular   cant*a*   ved*e*   dorm*e*

                plural   cant*ano*   ved*ono*   dorm*ono*

(9)

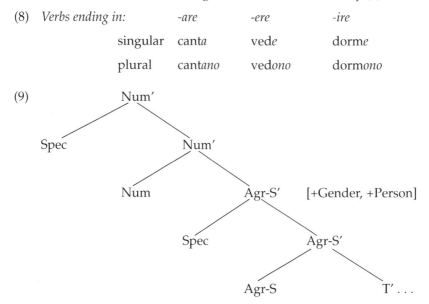

If it is true that Number c-selects Gender/Person in Italian, and that FCs cannot c-select categories which do not exist, it follows that Number will appear later than Gender and Person in the acquisition of Italian. The comprehension data, which are above chance, show that Italians aged 2;6 have Number in their grammars, and since performance on Number-inflected forms is somewhat low, we might argue that they do not *access* parameter-strings containing Number whenever necessary. But the data is not as simple as this: at the same time *verbal* Number appears to not be mastered, *noun plurals* have been mastered. Caselli *et al.*'s subjects scored 89% for production and 78% for comprehension of plural nouns; Leonard *et al.*'s control subjects scored 89.3% on production and 88.9% on comprehension for noun plurals. Differences between singular/plural forms were not significant this time. If Number hasn't been mastered in the grammar at 2;6, why is it showing up regularly and appropriately in noun plurals?

It is pretty self-evident that nominal Number has a clearer semantic status than verbal Number. People tend to think of 'plurality' as a property of nouns rather than abstract verb agreement. Booij (1993) analyses noun plurals as *inherent inflection*, and verbal Number as *contextual inflection*. Inherent inflection affects the semantics of its stem, e.g. 'Lynda's teddy bear/bears', whereas contextual inflection does not, e.g. 'I wear/she wears green pyjamas'. The semantic strength of noun plurals is clearly higher than that of verbal Number Agreement affixes. To say 'She wear green pyjamas' results in ungrammaticality, but no meaning change whatsoever.[2]

In Italian, where the subject is overt, its number marking will make Number agreement on the verb semantically redundant. Where the subject is covert (pro), its referent may be retrieved from the context, and Number on the verb is pragmatically redundant. Therefore, children who have not mastered verbal Number can still parse their input successfully, and generate structures which adults in turn can understand. But this only works for verbal Number. Children who have not mastered noun plurals will be far more likely to misinterpret what is said to them and to be difficult to understand, since noun plurals are needed fairly frequently in speech. While verbal Number errors may be *offset* to an extent by semantic and pragmatic cues, this is not the case for noun plurals: we might say that noun plurals are higher in *cue strength* than verbal Number affixes.

So, while the genetic algorithm model of parameter-setting predicts that verbal Number may not always be successfully *activated* in production and comprehension processing, the Competition Model predicts that noun plurals will be acquired faster than verbal Number inflections. The important point is that neither model on its own accounts for all the data on Italian Number: the GA model does not explain why noun plurals are mastered earlier (but the CM does); and the CM does not explain why Gender/Person Agreement, being as redundant as Number, is acquired earlier, nor why Number is only projected some of the time (but assumptions about c-selection and parameter value competition do).

The Functional Category Cueing model, bringing elements of both models together, is able to explain the data. We assume that Number is *available* in grammars at this stage; but it is not *activated* as strongly as grammars with Tense, Gender or Person due to c-selection constraints; it is not *activated* so strongly for verbal Number relative to noun plurals due to lower cue strength; and it is not *activated* all the time, as parameters are not set instantaneously, but after a period of competition between competing parameter stems.

Notes

1. This paper is a shorter version of one of the same title presented at the Child Language Seminar at UCNW in March 1994. It was written whjile the author was undertaking doctoral research, supported by ESRC studentship R00429234311 and supervised by Dr Susan Edwards and Prof Paul Fletcher.
2. Note that nominal Number Agreement between nouns and adjectives, which also takes place in Italian, is a case of contextual inflection, since the meaning of the adjective is not altered, and is semantically redundant, since Number is marked on the noun. The CM predicts that Number marking on adjectives should be acquired later/slower than noun plurals; unfortunately both elecitation studies looked only a Gender agreement on adjectives, so there is no data bearing on this prediction. However, Casselli *et al.* (1993) found a production rate of 75% and 81% for contextual plural Agreement on *Determiners* 'i' and 'le' — which shows strikingly similar percentages to verbal plural agreement production (80%); similar results are described by Leonard *et al.*, (1993:23) for Leonard *et al.*'s (1992) group.

References

Aksu-Koc, A. and Slobin, D. (1985) The acquisition of Turkish. In D. Slobin (ed.) *The Crosslinguistic Study of Language Acquisition* (pp.838–78). Hillsdale, NJ: Erlbaum.

Aldridge, M., Borsley, R. and Clack, S. (1994) The acquisition of Welsh clause structure. Paper presented at the LAGB meeting, Middlesex University.

Aoun, J. (1986) *Generalised Binding*. Dordrecht: Foris.

Baker, M. (1988) *Incorporation: A Theory of Grammatical Function Changing*. Chicago: University Of Chicago Press.

Bates, E., MacWhinney, B., Caselli, C., Devescovi, A., Natale, F. and Venva, V. (1984) A cross-sectional study of the development of sentence interpretation strategies. *Child Development* 55, 341–54.

Berwick, R. (1985) *The Acquisition of Syntactic Knowledge*. Cambridge, MA: MIT Press.

Booij, G. (1993) Against split morphology. In G. Booij and J. van Marle (eds.) *Yearbook of Morphology 1993*, 27–50. Dordrecht: Kluwer.

Borer, H. (1984) *Parametric Syntax*. Dordrecht: Foris.

Caselli, M., Leonard, L., Volterra, V. and Campanoli, M. (1993) Toward mastery of Italian morphology: A cross-sectional study. *Journal of Child Language* 20, 377–94.

Chomsky, N. (1991) Some notes on economy of derivation and representation. In R. Friedin (ed.) *Principles and Parameters in Comparative Grammar* (pp.417–59). Cambridge, MA: MIT Press.

— (1993) A minimalist program for linguistic theory. In K. Hale and S. Keyser (eds) *The View from Building 20: Essays in Linguistics in Honor of Sylvain Bromberger* (pp.1–52). Cambridge, MA: MIT Press.

Clahsen, H. (1991) *Child Language and Developmental Dysphasia: Linguistic Studies of the Acquisition of German*. Amsterdam: Benjamins.

Clancy, P. (1985) The acquisition of Japanese. In D. Slobin (ed.) *The Crosslinguistic Study of Language Acquisition* (pp.373–524). Hillsdale, NJ: Erlbaum.

Clark, R. (1990) Papers on learnability and natural selection. *Technical Reports in Formal and Computational Linguistics* 1, University of Geneva.

— (1992) The selection of syntactic knowledge. *Language Acquisition* 2, 85–149.

Clark, R. and Roberts, I. (1993) A computational model of language learnability and language change. *Linguistic Inquiry* 24, 299–346.

Collins, C. (1994) Economy of derivation and the generalised proper binding condition. *Linguistic Inquiry* 25, 45–61.

Fortesque, M. (1984) *West Greenlandic*. Beckenham: Croom Helm.

Fukuda, S. E. and Fukuda, S. (1994) Familial language impairment in Japanese: A linguistic investigation. *McGill Working Papers in Linguistics* 10, 150–77.

Fukui, N. (1986) A theory of category projection and its applications. PhD thesis, MIT.

— (1988) Deriving the differences between English and Japanese: a case study in parametric syntax. *English Linguistics* 5, 249–70.

Gibson, E. and Wexler, K. (1994) Triggers. *Linguistic Inquiry* 25, 407–54.

Guasti, M. (1993) Verb syntax in Italian child grammar: finite and non-finite verbs. *Language Acquisition* 3, 1–40.

Hernandez, A., Bates, E. and Avila, L. (1994) On-line sentence interpretation in Spanish-English bilinguals: What does it mean to be 'in between'? *Applied Psycholinguistics* 15, 417–46.

Hyams, N. (1984) Semantically based child grammars: Some empirical inadequacies. *Papers and Reports on Child Language Development* 23, 58–65.

Klima, E. and Bellugi, U. (1966) Syntactic regularities in the speech of children. In J. Lyons and R. Wales (eds) *Psycholinguistic Papers*. Edinburgh: Edinburgh University Press.

Leonard, L., Bortolini, U., Caselli, M., McGregor, K. and Sabbadini, L. (1992) Morphological deficits in children with specific language impairment: The status of features in the underlying grammar. *Language Acquisition* 2, 151–79.

Leonard, L., Bortolini, U., Caselli, M. and Sabbadini, L. (1993) The use of articles by Italian-speaking children with SLI. *Clinical Linguistics and Phonetics* 7, 19–28.

Leonard, L., Sabbadini, L., Leonard, J. and Volterra, V. (1987) Specific language impairment in children: A cross-linguistic study. *Brain and Language* 32, 233–52.

MacWhinney, B. (1989) Competition and teachability. In M. Rice and R. Schiefelbusch (eds) *The Teachability of Language* (pp.63–104). Baltimore: Brookes.

MacWhinney, B. and Bates, E. (eds) (1989) *The Crosslinguistic Study of Sentence Processing*. Cambridge: Cambridge University Press.

Madeira, A. (1993) Inflected infinitival clauses in Portuguese. Paper presented at the Autumn LAGB, UCNW, Wales.

McDonald, J. (1989) Determinants of the acquisition of cue-category mappings. In B. MacWhinney and E. Bates (eds) *The Crosslinguistic Study of Sentence Processing*. Cambridge: Cambridge University Press.

Ouhalla, J. (1991) *Functional Categories and Parametric Variation*. London: Routledge.

Pina, F. (1984) Teorias psico-soiolinguisticos y su aplicacion a la acquisicion del Espanol como lengua materna. Madrid: Siglo XXI.

Pizzuto, E. and Caselli, M. (1992) The acquisition of Italian morphology: Implications for models of language development. *Journal of Child Language* 19, 491–588.

— (1993) The acquisition of Italian morphology: A reply to Hyams. *Journal of Child Language* 20, 707–12.

Platzack, C. (1990) A grammar without functional categories: A syntactic study of early Swedish child language. Ms, Lund University.

Radford, A. (1987) The acquisition of the complementiser system. *Bangor Research Papers in Linguistics* 2, 55–76.

— (1990) *Syntactic Theory and the Acquisition of English Syntax*. Oxford: Blackwell.

Radford, A. and Aldridge, M. (1987) The acquisition of the Inflection system. In W. Lorscher and R. Schulze (eds) *Perspectives on Language Performance* (pp.1289–1309). Tubingen: Verlag.

Ritter, E. (1993) Where's Gender? *Linguistic Inquiry* 24, 795–803.

Shaer, B. (1989) Mood, Tense, and the Eskimo verb. Ms, Department of Linguistics, McGill University, Montreal.

Smoczynska, M. (1985) The acquisition of Polish. In D. Slobin (ed.) *The Crosslinguistic Study of Language Acquisition*. Hillsdale, NJ: Erlbaum.

Taylor, C. M. (1995a) Functional category cueing and imitation effects. PhD Thesis, University of Reading.

— (1995b) Negative morphemes in aphasia: Comments on Bebout (1993). *Clinical Linguistics and Phonetics* 9.

Tsimpli, I-M. (1991) On the maturation of functional categories. *UCL Working Papers in Linguistics* 3, 123–48.

— (1992) Functional categories and maturation: The prefunctional stage of language acquisition. PhD Thesis, UCL, London.

Weissenborn, J. (1988) The acquisition of clitic object pronouns and word order in French: syntax or morphology? Ms, Max Plank Institut Fur Psycholinguistik, Nijmegen.

Wexler, K. (1993) Optional infinitives, head movement, and the economy of derivations in child grammar. In N. Hornstein and D. Lightfoot (eds) *Verb Movement* (pp.305–50). Cambridge: Cambridge University Press.

Wexler, K. and Manzini, R. (1987) Parameters and learnability in binding theory. In T. Roeper and E. Williams (eds) *Parameter Setting*. Dordrecht: Reidel.

15 Language Modularity and Grammatical Specific Language Impairment in Children

HEATHER K. J. VAN DER LELY

Introduction

The investigations into specific language impairment (SLI) in children aim to characterize the nature of their disorder and in doing so provide particular insight into the issues of the modularity and domain specificity of language and the mechanisms of language acquisition. This is because differential functioning of language and cognitive abilities which is not apparent in normally developing children can be revealed in SLI children.

Language modularity

It is a contentious issue as to how the human mind is organized. However, how language is processed and represented in the brain has implications for theories of the underlying nature of SLI in children.

One view of the organisation of the mind suggests that language is 'non-modular', and may, or may not, be domain specific. Within this view, language processing relies on similar mechanisms to those used throughout the brain (Bates, 1995; Bates, Dale & Thal, 1993). Thus, it would be predicted that if a child was impaired in language then this should cause problems across all linguistic (and possibly non-linguistic) processing which rely on similar mechanisms.

Alternatively, the human mind may be viewed in terms of a distinction between the *central system* responsible for rational thought and the *fixation of beliefs,* and a number of modular input systems which feed the central system (Fodor, 1983). Fodor claims that the language faculty is one such modular system. Modules are domain specific, informationally encapsulated, fast, mandatory, subserved by specific neural architecture and subject to idiosyncratic pathological breakdown (Fodor, 1983). Domain specificity refers to the requirement that modules deal exclusively with a single information type. The neural specificity of the architecture may be taken to be genetically determined (innate) and therefore largely invariant across the species. Not all aspects of language fit into the definition of a module; for example, pragmatic inference and the storage of lexical-conceptual representations may be viewed as part of the central system, where as syntax, morphology and phonology are seen as part of the language module (Chomsky, 1986; Sperber & Wilson, 1986; Smith & Tsimpli, 1991, 1994).

Within this latter view of the organisation of language in the brain, it can be predicted that the SLI children's deficit may effect both the central system and the modular language system. Alternatively, the deficit could affect just modular language functioning. It is this narrow view that I shall be putting forward in this chapter; that is, SLI children suffer from a *modular language deficit*. Thus, it would be predicted that differential language functioning should be evident in SLI children. That is, particularly impaired performance should be found for modular language functions (such as, marking grammatical tense) but not for non-modular central language functions (such as pragmatic inference or lexical knowledge).

SLI in children

It is now well recognized that SLI in children is a heterogeneous disorder. This chapter is concerned with the investigations of a sub-group of 'Grammatical SLI' children who have a persistent and disproportionate impairment in the grammatical comprehension and expression of language. The groups is characterised by a similar linguistic profile. I do not claim that Grammatical SLI is, necessarily, an autonomous sub-group from all other SLI sub-groups, but I propose that the Grammatical SLI children are homogeneous *within* the sub-group.

The aims of this chapter are, first, to summarize the findings from a series of investigations into this sub-group of SLI children; secondly, to consider how far current theories of the underlying deficit in SLI can account for the data from Grammatical SLI children.

Grammatical SLI children: Background characteristics

The sub-group, classified as having a persisting SLI, were aged between 9;3–12;10 (years; months). The SLI children had been diagnosed by speech and language therapists as having severe and persistent difficulties with language development as measured on standardised tests of language abilities. That is, their scores fell more than –1.5 sd below that expected for their chronological age. In addition, the children were characterised as having a disproportionate deficit in morpho-syntactic expression and comprehension of language over and above any 'general' language impairment in other areas of language (e.g. lexical-semantic knowledge of single words). The SLI children were matched to a group of 12 normally developing children (Language Ability (LA1) controls, aged, 5;5–6;4) on tests of aspects of morpho-syntactic abilities and to two groups (the LA2 controls (aged 6;5–7;4) and the LA3 controls (aged 7;5–8;9)) on tests of single word receptive and expressive vocabulary development. A summary of the subject's details can be found in Table 15.1.

Table 15.1 Subject details: Chronological ages and raw scores from the four standardised tests used for matching purposes

	Subjects				
	SLI children (N = 12) Mean (sd)	LA1 controls (N = 12) Mean (sd)	LA2 controls (N = 12) Mean (sd)	LA3 controls (N = 12) Mean (sd)	Summary of analysis between groups
Chronological age	11;2 (1;1)	5;9 (0;4)	6;11 (0;4)	7;11 (0;5)	
Range	9;3-12:10	5;5-6:4	6;5-7:4	7;5-8:9	
TROG	13.08 (1.78)	14.41 (8.56)	16.00 (1.75)	17.33 (1.23)	LA1 = SLI< (LA2 = LA3)
GC-ITPA	20.00 (3.56)	21.25 (3.16)	26.25 (4.08)	28.91 (2.19)	LA1 = SLI< (LA2 = LA3)
BPVS	78.83 (8.93)	56.25 (8.91)	71.67 (9.71)	80.00 (9.62)	LA1 < SLI= (LA2 < LA3)
NV-BAS	17.91 (1.17)	15.67 (1.61)	17.17 (1.27)	17.50 (0.90)	LA1 < SLI= (LA2 = LA3)

(Note: TROG = Test of reception of grammar (Bishop, 1983); GC-ITPA = Grammatical closure sub- test from the Illinois Test of Psycholinguistic Abilities (Kirk *et al.*, 1968); BPVS = British picture vocabulary scale (Dunn *et al.*, 1982); NV-BAS = Naming Vocabulary from the British Ability Scales (Elliott *et al.*, 1978)).

Children were excluded from the group if they had social-emotional abnormalities or 'semantic- pragmatic' SLI (Bishop & Adams, 1989), or if they had articulatory dyspraxia, a severe phonological disorder, omitted final consonants (regardless of the grammatical context) and/or were partially unintelligible.

The findings from a preliminary investigation into familiar aggregation of language impairment in these Grammatical SLI children was consistent with an autosomal dominant genetic inheritance underlying their disorder (see van der Lely & Stollwerck, in press).

Grammatical SLI Children: Findings from Previous Investigations

Inflectional morphology: 1. Regular and irregular past tense marking

I shall first present preliminary evidence of regular and irregular past tense marking in the Grammatical SLI children's expressive language. In collaboration with Michael Ullman and Steven Pinker the children's judgement of past tense forms has also been investigated (van der Lely & Ullman, in preparation).

Evidence for the SLI children's and LA1 controls' marking of past tense on regular verbs (e.g. *jump-jumped*) and irregular verbs (e.g. *swim-swam*) was obtained from a narrative based on a picture book ('Frog where are you?'). Detailed transcriptions were made from a high quality DAT tape recording. Auxiliaries and past participles were not included in the analysis. Verbs were also excluded if they were followed by a word starting with a 't' and there was any ambiguity as to whether the past tense had been marked on the verb.

An initial analysis was carried out on the total number of verb types and tokens used in the narrative (see Table 15.2). The overall mean number of verb types and tokens used by the two groups did not differ. In addition, the two groups were found to use a similar number of regular and irregular verbs in past tense contexts. The total number of past tense errors was calculated as a proportion of the total number of verbs used in a past tense context; i.e. where a stem form was used for a regular or irregular verb in a past tense context, or a regular *ed* morpheme was affixed to an irregular verb. It can be seen from Table 15.2 that the SLI children made proportionally significantly more overall total errors on both the regular and irregular verbs than the LA1 controls. The SLI children made approximately 25% errors for the regular and irregular past tense marking whereas the LA1 controls made hardly any errors at all for the regular verbs (0.7–0.9%) and only 5–8% errors for the irregular verbs. For the irregular verbs the SLI children's errors were almost equally divided between stem errors (8–10%) and overregularisation errors (e.g. *swimmed; falled*) (9–12%).

Table 15.2 Spontaneous speech analysis: Summary of the mean scores for regular and irregular verbs for the SLI children and the LA1 controls

	SLI children Mean (SD)	LA1 controls Mean (SD)
Overall verb total		
Types	28.58 (5.66)	29.33 (5.35)
Tokens	55.33 (16.92)	59.33 (18.00)
Irregular past tense contexts		
Types	10.25 (2.80)	7.76 (4.61)
Tokens	18.25 (5.68)	14.17 (9.15)
Regular past tense contexts		
Types	8.00 (1.81)	6.91 (5.04)
Tokens	12.67 (4.07)	9.83 (7.19)
% Regular errors (Total)		
Types	24.57 (28.23)	0.91 (2.87)
Tokens	23.49 (29.33)	0.72 (2.26)
% Irregular errors (Total)		
Types	25.32 (15.57)	8.13 (9.32)
Tokens	19.27 (14.93)	5.29 (6.45)
% Irregular Stem errors:		
Types	10.26 (13.51)	2.37 (5.27)
Tokens	8.32 (11.88)	1.67 (3.55)
% Irregular Overregularisations		
Types	12.48 (9.72)	2.72 (5.09)
Tokens	9.31 (8.32)	1.94 (3.94)

If we look at 'no tense' marking, rather that the total number of errors for the irregular and regular verbs for the SLI children, we find considerably more no tense marking errors for the regular verbs than the irregular verbs (approximately 24% vs 10% respectively). In contrast, the LA controls show more stem errors (i.e. zero marking) for the irregular verbs, whereas they virtually do not make errors on regular verbs. The Group X Verb type interaction was approaching significance ($F(1,20) = 3.79$, $p = 0.066$). T-tests confirmed a significant difference between the groups for the stem errors on the regular verbs (Types, $t(20) = 2.77$, $p = 0.011$; Tokens, $t(20) = 2.57$, $p = 0.018$) but the difference did not reach significance for the irregular stem errors.

To summarise: (1) In approximately 75% of past tense context SLI children mark past tense correctly. (2) The SLI children make significantly more overall errors than younger children matched on language abilities on both regular and irregular verbs. This finding concurs with Bishop (in press) who also found errors for both regular and irregular past tense marking. (3) The SLI children do not mark past tense on main verbs approximately 25% of the time for regular verbs and 10% of the time for irregular verbs. (4) The SLI children make significantly more stem errors on regular verbs than the LA controls who virtually do not make errors on regular verbs. (5) Approximately 12% overregularisations of irregular verbs in past tense contexts were made by the SLI children. This level of overregularisation is considerably more than the rate of overregularisation which may be used by children developing normally at certain early periods of their development. For example, Marcus, Pinker, Ullman, Hollander, Rosen & Xu, (1992) quote a rate of between 2–5% for some of the children which they study.

The findings indicate that the SLI children do not obligatorily mark past tense in sentences and may overgeneralise the infinitive form to past tense contexts. Their deficit, however, appears to be more pronounced for regular verbs than for irregular verbs. From these data we do not know whether the SLI children's stem errors are performance errors or whether, for the SLI children, tense does not have to be obligatorily marked, as suggested by Rice, Wexler & Cleave (in press). The results of a grammatical judgement task of regular and irregular words and nonce words in past tense contexts provide further insight into this issue. In this chapter, I shall only report the results from the real verbs.

In the judgement task the children heard a lead in sentence containing the verb in the present tense. This was followed by a sentence with the verb in a past tense context. The verb in this second sentence was given in three forms on different occasions, i.e. the stem form, the correct past tense form and an overregularized form for irregular verbs and a pseudo irregular form for the regular verbs. For example, *Every day I swim a mile. Just like every day, yesterday I swim/swam/swimmed a mile. Every day I walk home. Just like every day, yesterday I walk/wok/walked home* (see Table 15.3). The child's task was to judge whether the verb form in the second sentence was good/correct or not good/incorrect. Table 15.3 shows that the SLI children primarily correctly accept irregular and regular past tense forms and reject irregularisations of regular verbs in past tense contexts. However, in contrast to the LA controls, they incorrectly accept stem forms and overregularisations of irregular verbs in past tense contexts. The results are consistent with their production of verbs in past tense contexts. The findings provide further support for the claim that SLI children do not obligatorily mark tense and overgeneralise the infinitival or present verb forms (which are generally indistinguishable in English from the stem forms) to past tense contexts.

Table 15.3 The SLI children and LA1 control children's judgements for the three verb forms for the regular and irregular verbs

Verb form	Example of verb form	SLI children's judgements	LA control's judgements
Irregular verb form	*Swam*	YES	YES
	Wok	NO	NO
Stem form	*Swim*	YES	NO
	Walk	YES	NO
Regular form	*Swimmed*	YES	NO
	Walked	YES	YES

Subject-verb agreement: Elicitation task

Each of the SLI children were asked to list 10 things their father or mother did in the mornings when they went to school. The child's responses were recorded using a DAT Sony tape recorder. As is characteristically found for SLI children, this group also made a large number of omissions of obligatory third person agreement 's' on the verb. As a group, they made 60% verb type and 49% verb token agreement omissions. All except one child had over 20% agreement errors.

Summary

The grammatical SLI children show a significant impairment in inflectional morphology for subject verb agreement marking. The pattern of inflectional morphological impairment for this older group of English speaking SLI children concur with the data from previous investigations of younger English and German SLI children (Bishop, in press; Clahsen, 1989, 1991; Leonard, 1989; Leonard, McGregor & Allen, 1992; Rice & Oetting, 1991). However, the Grammatical SLI children's problems extend beyond inflectional morphology and also affect their syntax.

Theta role assignment

The SLI children's problems with theta role assignment have been revealed in a picture pointing task in which the children have to interpret reversible sentences, i.e. sentences in which the lexical items do not provide semantic or pragmatic cues as to their thematic roles (see van der Lely, 1993 for full details of this investigation).

Surprisingly, even in the interpretation of simple active, transitive sentences these SLI children made approximately 8% errors, assigning the theme to the first noun phrase (NP), and the agent to the second NP. However, it is with full passive (e.g. *The boy is pinched by the girl*) and unambiguously short passive sentences (e.g. *The car is being hit*) that the SLI children make a substantial number of errors. As a group they made 40% errors on the full passives and 33% errors on the short unambiguous passive sentences. Thus, they made almost as many errors interpreting the full passive sentences as they do when attempting to mark subject verb agreement in their expressive language.

Grammatical SLI children's problems with theta roles are also evident in their expressive language. Occasional omissions of obligatory arguments are found in their utterances. For example in the narrative discourse discussed above, SLI 7 said the following: *The boy caught a fish- a frog- and he put (0) in the jar.* Thus, it appears that the SLI children's problems with theta roles are evident in both their comprehension and expression of language. Any explanation for the SLI children's deficit must therefore take this into account.

Reference assignment to pronouns and reflexives in sentences

Grammatical SLI children's syntactic problems are also apparent when reference assignment to pronouns (*him/her*) and anaphors, such as reflexives (*himself/herself*), is dependent on syntactic knowledge of locality condition in the binding of reflexives and pronouns. This syntactic knowledge has been characterized within the linguistic theory of Government and Binding (Chomsky, 1981, 1986) by the Binding Principles A & B respectively. In the sentences in (1) and (2) below it can be seen that the reflexive must refer to Grannie and not Minni the Minx, where as the pronoun must not refer to 'Grannie' but can refer to Minni the Minx.

(1) Minni the Minx$_i$ says Grannie$_j$ is pinching herself$_{*i/j}$

(2) Minni the Minx$_i$ says Grannie$_j$ is pinching her$_{i/*j}$

An experiment involving a sentence-picture judgement task (based on Chien & Wexler, 1990) was undertaken to investigate the Grammatical SLI children's knowledge of the lexical and syntactic properties of pronouns and reflexives. It was found that if the SLI children were given a picture showing Grannie pinching herself and asked if sentence (2) (spoken by the experimenter) was correct, they performed at chance. The SLI children failed to reject the mismatch around 40% of the time. When the picture showed Minni the Minx pinching herself and sentence (1) was spoken, the children failed to correctly identify the mismatch 50% of the time. In this latter case the lexical properties of *herself* were correct and only the syntactic condition (principle A) was violated. That is, a self-oriented action was depicted, but the picture incorrectly showed a non-local antecedent carrying out the action. In contrast to the SLI children's inability to use knowledge of the syntactic structure to assign reference to the pronoun and reflexive, they showed a good ability to use lexical-semantic cues, such as semantic gender, to assign coreference and their performance did not differ from the three groups of LA control children (see van der Lely & Stollwerck, 1993 for further details).

The Underlying Nature of SLI in Children

The evidence presented above, in which aspects of inflectional morphology and syntactic language abilities were investigated in a group of Grammatical SLI children has indicted that these children have a significant deficit in both of these areas of language. I shall now attempt to account for these data within current theories of the underlying deficit causing SLI in children.

I shall first consider the auditory perceptual limitations hypothesis (Leonard, 1989; Leonard, McGregor & Allen, 1992). Leonard has based his theory primarily on the expressive language of SLI children of 2–6 years of age. Recently Leonard and his colleagues have supplemented data from English speaking SLI children with data from Italian (Leonard, Bartolini, Caselli, McGregor & Sabbadini, 1992) and Hebrew (Dromi, Leonard & Shteiman, 1993). Leonard puts forward that, due to a general perceptual deficit, SLI children have difficulties in discriminating 'low-phonetic substance' or non-salient morphemes, such as the 's' in plurals and subject–verb agreement for third person singular, and the 't/d' which marks past tense on regular verbs. Leonard argues that these elements are particularly vulnerable to loss and that extra resources are needed to perceive them. As a consequence of this, processing resources are used up from the SLI children's already limited resources. Thus, additional operations cannot be performed adequately such as building morphological paradigms. Note, Leonard's hypothesis tacitly assumes that the deficit is a non- modular language deficit.

Leonard's proposal can account for the subject verb agreement errors and the frequent omissions of regular past tense marking which were found in the data for the grammatical SLI children. However, vowel changes, which are perceptually salient, constitute the majority of phonological differences between the irregular verb stems and their past tense forms. Thus, it is difficult to see how a perceptual deficit and limited processing resources can account for these errors. For the same reason, Leonard's proposal can not account for the SLI children's acceptance of irregular stem forms in past tense contexts. It is also difficult to see how the auditory perceptual hypothesis can account for the syntactic deficits that have been found for the Grammatical SLI children, such as their difficulties in assigning thematic roles to noun phrases and in determining the reference of pronouns and reflexives in sentences.

The remaining hypotheses characterising SLI in children I shall consider assume a specific modular language deficit underlies SLI. The first of these modular hypothesis was proposed by Gopnik (1990) and Gopnik & Crago (1991) and was developed to account for data from her investigations into a large family of 30 members of whom half had a language impairment. Gopnik (1990) proposed that the underlying deficit in the SLI family could be characterized by a lack of morpho-syntactic features, such as tense, aspect, gender and number.

This theory may account for the grammatical SLI children's subject–verb agreement errors. This is because knowledge of features, such as the number and person of the noun, are required for the correct agreement inflection on the verb. In addition the missing feature hypothesis can account for the general problem the grammatical SLI children have with marking tense with both irregular and regular verbs and their acceptance of the stem verb forms in past tense contexts: without adequate specification of the tense feature, tense will not be appropriately realise. However, as with the auditory perceptual deficit hypothesis, the missing feature hypothesis is not consistent with the disproportionate deficit the grammatical SLI children have with subject–verb agreement; with the assignment of thematic roles in reversible passive sentences; nor with the impairment in reference assignment to reflexives and pronouns within sentences.

The third hypothesis I shall consider is Clahsen's (1989, 1991) Grammatical Agreement deficit hypothesis. This hypothesis was based on his investigations of a sub-group of German speaking SLI children. Clahsen put forward that SLI in children is caused by a selective deficit with agreement in an otherwise intact grammatical system. Thus, within Government and Binding Theory (Chomsky, 1981, 1986), this can be interpreted as meaning that features of AGR (gender, person, number) will not be correctly realised.

It is evident from the data from the Grammatical SLI children that we can not say that AGR or agreement is *missing*. If this were so, we would not expect the SLI children to achieve around 50% correct subject–verb agreement. However, a weaker view of this hypothesis does correctly predict the particular difficulties the SLI children have with subject–verb agreement. Unfortunately, it is more difficult to see how this hypothesis can account for the other difficulties shown to exist with the grammatical SLI children's language, such as their problems with tense, theta role assignment and anaphoric reference in sentences. The agreement hypothesis as put forward by Clahsen (1989) would not predict any problems in these areas of syntax. It is evident that the particular deficit in the syntax and morphology shown by the grammatical SLI children is broader than either the missing feature or agreement hypotheses.

In an earlier work (van der Lely, 1994) I proposed that the expressive and receptive language of grammatical SLI children could be accounted for by a deficit in dependent structural relationships between constituents. I shall refer to this as a Representational Deficit for Dependent Relationships (RDDR). A dependent relationship between representations may be found, for example, with subject–verb agreement when the inflectional form of the verb is dependent on the syntactic relationship between the noun phrase and the verb, and the grammatical number and person of the noun. In sentence comprehension, the assignment of theta roles to a noun phrase is dependent on a combination of the verb's lexical properties and the noun's syntactic relationship to the verb (i.e. whether it is the subject NP or object NP). It is only when 'knowledge' of such a relationship between structures is required, that is when lexical, pragmatic or general world knowledge is insufficient, that SLI children's impaired comprehension is apparent.

Whilst the RDDR proposal captures the deficits shown by grammatical SLI children, a more specific linguistic characterisation is desirable if it is to be a useful notion through which to explore SLI in children. There are clearly similarities with the notion of the RDDR proposal and Clahsen's missing agreement hypothesis in that the RDDR also suggest that it is the dependent relationships between constituents which are problematic for SLI children. However, the agreement deficit hypothesis proposed by Clahsen (1989) appears to be too narrow a linguistic characterisation to account for the findings from English speaking SLI children. As already mentioned, the agreement hypothesis, for example, can not account for the deficits found with inflectional marking of tense, the assignment of theta roles, or the problems with the interpretation of pronouns and reflexives in sentences. Thus, a broader characterisation is required.

Van der Lely (1994) proposed that a deficit in the area of 'government' or 'locality' (Chomsky, 1986; Manzini & Wexler, 1987) which specifies the syntactic relationships between constituents can account for the data from SLI children. This proposal captures the notion of the RDDR proposal and can account for the deficits in tense, theta role assignment, and coreference of pronouns and anaphors in sentences. However, a deficit in government would also predict that SLI children would have problems with both constituent-internal and sequential word order among many other deficits. Word order problems are not generally cited as a characteristic of SLI children's language, although they do occasionally occur. In the data cited above from the narrative discourse, a very obvious word order error by subject SLI 7 occurred: *Bees the nest* = 'The bees nest'.

The possibility that SLI children achieve correct word order by other means can not be ruled out, e.g. theta roles (e.g. Agent, Theme) may be mapped directly onto NP positions (first NP, second NP). It is interesting to note that SLI children have a tendency to omit phrasal and sentential constituents when two or more elements are required and produce few phrases with more than two elements (Cromer, 1981; Fletcher, Ingham & Kirby, 1992; Leonard, 1989). Words which have (central system) semantic support such as lexical constituents may be more likely to be correctly realised that those which rely to a greater extent on syntactic representation such as functional constituents. Thus, more general (central system) learning mechanisms may enable SLI children to achieve the level of linguistic functioning that they do. It would appear that such a possible learning strategy is insufficient for the SLI child to reach adult language functioning.

I conclude that whilst the agreement hypothesis is too narrow, it is likely that a deficit in government is too broad. It seems more plausible that a linguistic characterisation of grammatical SLI lies somewhere in between agreement and government. It is clear that there is much work to be done to provide an adequate linguistic characterisation of the RDDR proposal. Further research in this area may not only provide a more adequate characterisation of SLI in children but may facilitate greater specification of the modularity of language.

The findings so far from Grammatical SLI children are consistent with a modular, domain specific defect. That is, particular problems are found with (arguably) modular language functions but not language abilities which primarily rely on the central system. Deficits were found in areas of syntax (Tense, Theta theory, Binding Principles) but not in the ability to use semantic-lexical properties of constituents (e.g. semantic gender) to facilitate interpretation of sentences. Thus, the language characteristics of Grammatical SLI children provide support for the modularity of language theory.

References

Bates, E. (1993) Modularity, domain specificity and the development of language. *Technical Report, 9305, Project in Cognitive Neuroscience*. University of California, San Diego.

Bates, E., Dale, P. and Thal, D. (1995) Individual differences and their implications for theories of language development. In P. Fletcher & B. MacWhinney (eds) *Handbook of Child Language*. Oxford: Basil Blackwell.

Bishop, D. V. M. (1983) *Test of Reception of Grammar*. Manchester University.

— (in press) Grammatical errors in specific language impairment: Competence or performance limitations? *Applied Psycholinguistics*.

Bishop, D. V. M. and Adams, C. (1989) Conversational characteristics of children with semantic-pragmatic disorder. 2: What features lead to a judgement of inappropriacy? *British Journal of Disorders of Communication* 24, 241–64

Chien, Y-C. and Wexler, K. (1990) Children's knowledge of locality conditions in binding as evidence for the modularity of syntax and pragmatics. *Language Acquisition*, 1, 225–95.

Chomsky, N. (1981) *Lectures on Government and Binding*. Dordrecht: Foris.

— (1986) *Knowledge of Language: Its Nature, Origin and Use*. NY: Praeger.

Clahsen, H. (1989) The grammatical characterisation of developmental dysphasia. *Linguistics* 27, 897–920.

— (1991) *Child Language and Developmental Dysphasia*. Amsterdam, Netherlands: John Bejamins Publishing Company.

Cromer, R. (1981) Hierarchical ordering disability and aphasic children. In P. Dale & D. Ingram (eds) *Child Language. An International Perspective*. Baltimore: Univ Press.

Dromi, E., Leonard, L. and Shteiman, M. (1993) The grammatical morphology of Hebrew-speaking children with specific language impairment: some competing hypotheses. *Journal of Speech and Hearing Research* 36, 760–71.

Dunn, L., Dunn, L., Whetton, C. and Pintilie, D., (1982) *The British Picture Vocabulary Scales*. Windsor: NFER-Nelson

Elliott, C., Murray, D. and Pearson, L. (1978) *British Ability Scales*. Windsor: NFER-Nelson

Fletcher, P., Ingham, R. and Kirby, G. (1992) The grammatical characterisation of specific language impairment: Theoretical and methodological issues. In I. Warburton & R. Ingham (eds) *Working Papers in General and Applied Linguistics*. Department of Linguistic Science, Reading University. UK: Reading, pp. 112–31.

Fodor, F. J. (1983) *The Modularity of Mind*. Cambridge, MA: MIT Press.

Gopnik, M. (1990) Feature Blindness: A case study. *Language Acquisition* 1, 139–64.

Gopnik, M. and Crago, M. (1991) Familial aggregation of a developmental language disorder, *Cognition* 39, 1–50.

Hurst, J., Baraister, M., Auger, E., Graham, F. and Norrell S. (1990) An extended family with an inherited speech disorder. *Developmental Medicine and Child Neurology* 32, 347–55.

Kirk, S., McCarthy J. and Kirk, W. (1968) *Illinois Test of Psycholinguistic Abilities*. Urbana, IL: Univ Press.

Leonard, L. B. (1989) Language learnability and specific language impairment in children. *Applied Psycholinguistics* 10, 179–202

Leonard, L., Bartolini, U., Caselli, C., McGregor, K. and Sabbadini, L. (1992) Morphological deficits in children with specific language impairment: The status of features in the underlying grammar. *Language Acquisition* 2, 151–79.

Leonard, L. McGregor, K. and Allen, G. (1992). Grammatical morphology and speech perception in children with specific language impairment. *Journal of Speech and Hearing Research* 35, 1076–1085.

Manzini, R. and Wexler, K. (1987) Parameters, binding theory, and learnability. *Linguistic Inquiry* 18, 413–44.

Marcus, G., Pinker, S., Ullman, M., Hollander, M., Rosen, J. and Xu, F. (1992) *Overregularisation in Language Acquisition. Monographs of the Society for Research in Child Development*. Series 228, 57, 4. University of Chicago Press.

Rice, M. and Oetting, J. (1991) Morphological deficits of SLI children: evaluation of number marking and agreement. Paper presented at *The Boston University Conference on Language Development*. October, 1991, Boston, MA.

Rice, M., Wexler, K. and Cleave, P. (in press) Specific language impairment as a period of extended optional infinitive. *Journal of Speech and Hearing Research*.

Smith, N. and Tsimpli, I. (1991) Linguistic Modularity? A case study of a 'savant' linguist. *Lingua* 84, 315–51.

— (1994) A specialist intelligence: The case of a polyglot savant. *University College London, Working Papers in Linguistics*, 5. London: Department of Phonetics and Linguistics, Univ. College London.

Sperber, D. and Wilson, D. (1986) *Relevance: Communication and Cognition*. Oxford: Blackwell.

Van der Lely, H. K. J. (1993) Specifically language impaired children and normally developing children: Different patterns of sentence comprehension. In J. Clibbens & B. Pendleton (eds) *Proceedings from The Child Language Seminar 1993*. University of Plymouth, England, pp. 59–80.

— (1994) Canonical linking rules: Forward vs Reverse linking in normally developing and specifically language impaired children. *Cognition* 51, 29–72.

Van der Lely, H. K. J. and Stollwerck, L. (in press) A grammatical specific language impairment in children: An Autosomal Dominant Inheritance? *Brain & Language.*

— (1993) Language modularity, Binding Theory and specifically language impaired children. Paper presented at *Generative Approaches to Language Acquisition, 1993* Durham University, UK. September 17-19, 1993.

Van der Lely, H. K. J. and Ullman, M. (in preparation) The computation of inflectional morphology in Grammatical specifically language impaired children.

16 Talking about Reading Strategies with Poor Readers: A Way of Increasing Student Control of the Learning Situation

JULIE WAIT

This paper focuses on the second of three in-depth case studies on individual poor readers. The central question was: To what extent can talk about reading strategies increase student control in learning to read? Shared reading sessions were undertaken with a nine-year-old girl over one term. Data collection methods included audio and video recording which was subsequently transcribed, and a tutor diary reflecting on interaction.

Data analysis of student and tutor behaviour indicated an overall increase in the student's control of the learning situation at critical moments during the reading sessions.

Introduction

The vast body of literature on assisting poor readers that has accumulated over the last few decades has been concerned almost exclusively with learners in situations in which they have little control over their learning. This literature has included particular instruction methods such as Direct Instruction (Engelmann & Bruner, 1983), Corrective Feedback (Rose *et al.*, 1982), Pause Prompt and Praise (McNaughton *et al.*, 1987) and Context Cuing (Mudre & McCormick, 1989). These approaches were based on behaviourist theory. As a peripatetic teacher of children with reading difficulties I found the teaching methods to be unsuitable as they were not flexible enough to serve individual needs.

Approaches of action researchers (Meek, 1983; Martin, 1989) have been more versatile. Above all the main strength in such studies has been the handing over of responsibility of learning to the student. Therefore, I decided to undertake a series of case-studies with children with reading difficulties which sought ways in which the learner could be given more control. In addition I aimed to collect systematic data to show the development of reading strategies within a broad framework.

From experience with poor readers, in particular an initial case study, I had found that there were a number of ways which increased the learner's control. Firstly, being able to choose the text was clearly a motivating factor. Secondly, negotiating the structure and form of assistance during reading practice. Thirdly, encouraging the student to talk about reading behaviour. The third of these seemed to have been largely ignored by other researchers so the main question that I asked was: To what extent can talk about reading strategies increase the student's control of the reading process? Three in-depth case-studies were undertaken and it is the second of these which is the focus of this report.

Case Study

Student's background

Alice, who was 9 years 10 months at the outset of the study, lived with her mother, her mother's fiancé and her younger half-brother. Her mother had literacy difficulties but the fiancé was able to offer support to both mother and daughter. Alice had had plenty of good literacy opportunities and owned many books. The children at Alice's school came from a wide variety of socio-economic backgrounds although families were mostly in the middle income bracket living in small privately-owned houses.

Reading

The school had recognised Alice's reading difficulties from a young age. According to the class teacher her reading was about two years behind the class average. She read with the classroom assistant most days and to the classteacher about twice a week. These books were graded and were mostly from reading schemes. She had access to other books during silent reading periods which were scheduled on a daily basis. Silent reading was done individually and Alice had also done some reading with a friend during breaktimes. However, overall the amount of shared reading which was student-led was minimal. She had also been given a small amount of structured teaching on a small group basis using multi-sensory methods.

Teacher viewpoint

The classteacher put emphasis on her level of confidence and how he had seen this change from his last close contact as her classteacher when she was seven. He considered that any individual reading practice was good for Alice and recognised the importance in her reading a variety of texts.

Parent viewpoint

Alice's mother and partner were interviewed at their home before the start of the study. Although they offered a supportive and caring environment Alice did not practise much reading at home. The parents were aware of a difference in Alice's attitude towards home and school reading. She was far more conscientious at school than at home. They had found her most willing to read in informal situations. However, they were encouraging only a narrow set of reading strategies with much emphasis on grapho-phonics and little on holistic methods.

Student viewpoint

Alice said that she liked the reading that she was doing with the classroom assistant. She said that at the start that she found the books interesting although by the end of the study she implied that she had tired of them. When asked what she did when she came to something in a book that she didn't know she said that she sought adult help. She said that she thought good readers would do the same.

Method

Organisation of shared reading sessions

I worked on an individual basis with Alice for three sessions of 40 minutes per week over eight weeks. The sessions, which were in addition to the usual reading practice, were devoted to the shared reading of a variety of texts. A special small room was used so that any interruptions and distractions could be kept to a minimum.

Shared reading texts

Alice chose all the texts that were read; none were imposed. They came from a variety of sources including the school library and books brought in from our homes. Fiction, poetry and information texts of varying levels of complexity were read. After selecting a book Alice chose the way in which it was shared. Generally, she preferred to take it in turns to read alternate pages. We did little simultaneous reading because she said she felt uncomfortable with that method.

Data collection

All vocal behaviour of student and tutor was transcribed from an audio and video recording. Relevant non-verbal behaviour was also noted in the transcription. Also I kept a diary which provided a record of personal reactions to the sessions.

Data Analysis

Reading strategies used were initially grouped under three main headings according to the types of knowledge they displayed:

1. Knowledge about Language

2. Bibliographic Knowledge

3. Knowledge about the World.

Talk about these types of knowledge was embedded in the ongoing interaction of each session. Categorisation of strategies under these headings was chosen as a means of illustrating the wide range of strategies that was influencing the student's reading. In relation to each heading I will discuss indications of increasing control.

Knowledge about language

Students make reference to a wide range of aspects of language during the reading process. In the first few sessions I became increasingly aware of the need to develop Alice's concept of rhyming. Experience of rhyme has been identified as an important contributory factor in learning to read. Children with reading difficulties invariably have problems with this aspect and studies have shown advantages of developing rhyming skills (e.g. Bryant & Bradley, 1985).

Rhyming

The dialogue focusing on rhyming that took place during the reading sessions suggested that Alice's understanding and application of rhyming gradually progressed. The data showed that she needed to gain from experience of listening to rhyme before taking a more active role in the reading of rhyme. I refer to a number of extracts to illustrate this progression.

After reading 'Mr Magnolia' in *Session 2*, I found she was not able to identify rhyming words. Even though I drew her attention to one word of a rhyming pair she was unable to find the other word:

Tutor: Newt rhymes with

Alice: rhymes with

T: rhymes with something that's not on that page (turns over)

A: He picks holes in his suit. I thought that (long pause)

T: Suit rhymes with newt, right?

A: Yes

T: and also with (long pause) boot.

Experience in listening to rhyme

In *Session 5* we had read a story that ended in a song. Alice was only able to identify the rhyming words after she had listened and followed the words of the song, thus matching letter patterns and sounds. As in the previous example Alice had not recognised that it was the words rather than the lines that rhymed. I read the song.

A: That line and them two (She points to correct lines)

T: That line and that line rhyme because the words that rhyme are:

A: Be and me

T: Me that's right.

In *Session 7* more difficult poems were shared. Alice was saying as well as locating the rhyming words.

By *Session 12* Alice was quite confident about finding rhyming words; she needed much less help in finding rhyming pairs than previously. She identified pairs such as come and hum; ball and call; hop and top quite independently.

Experiencing rhyme as a reader

Later on in *Session 12* Alice showed that she could detect rhyme when she was the reader. She read a poem about a city:

T: What do you think of that?

A: It's nice.

T: Nice poem, yeh. Any more rhyming there?

A: Kite and

T: You don't mean kite

A: Wings and sings.

T: Good girl

A: Bed and head.

In *Session 13* Alice was able to anticipate rhyming. She recognised rhyming in the first verse and explained that this meant there was likely to be rhyming in other verses.

In *Session 17* Alice demonstrated the ability to isolate rhyming words from a whole text without prompting; thus showing an increase in control over learning about reading rhyming words:

T: Anything else that makes it like poetry, not all poetry, but quite a bit of poetry?

A: Oh it always ends in the same letters like 'tin' and 'in' (she finds the appropriate words in the text as she says this).

Table 16.1 summarises these findings.

Table 16.1 Knowledge about language: Rhyming

Session	Behaviour Observed
2	Unable to identify rhyming pairs following tutor prompting
5, 7, 12	Able to identify rhyming pairs after tutor prompting when listening to rhyme
12	Able to identify rhyming pairs after tutor prompting when reading rhyme
17	Able to identify rhyming pairs unaided

Bibliographic knowledge

This refers to strategies in which the reader draws on knowledge about books. Much of this knowledge can be obtained from being read to rather than actually being the reader.

Using pictures

In *Session 4* Alice's reflection on miscues reveals that she was using pictures as a word-solving device:

A: shout

T: So what have you said? (pause) So why do you think you said 'shout?'

A: Because I thought she was shouting. (Alice points to the picture of the girl with her mouth open.)

In the diary I had noted that:

'the girl's mouth is nearly always open throughout the illustrations'.

From such discussion I realised that Alice used pictures as cues as she went along for word-solving. However, she rarely practised more complex skills such as using illustrations to predict the sequence of events and as a means of enriching background knowledge. My diary notes made reference to this point on several occasions.

During the early sessions I had made suggestions before reading such as 'Have a good look through'. However, Alice had tended not to preview stories from the pictures. This needed to be developed.

Progress in using pictures to preview a story was apparent in some of the later sessions. It occurred in *Session 13* during the reading of a poem and then later in *Session 21* when she looked through the pictures of 'The Sultan's Snakes' before reading. The snakes are hidden within each room. After a few pages Alice began to think aloud:

A: Might be snakes, might be snakes — all this might be snakes.(mm) Yeh, that might be a snake mmmm.

T: I think you've got the idea of the story, what the story is . . .

Then she predicted the events of the story from the pictures:

A: They escape

T: Yes

A: And he looks in the bin, they're all gone. They make a plate. . . .

Combining pictures and titles was a strategy that was talked about later in the same session when Alice chose to read 'The Topsy Turvey Story-book'. I encouraged her to predict the theme from the book and then look at the story and rhyme titles to develop useful background information (see Table 16.2).

Table 16.2 Bibliographic knowledge: Using pictures

Session	Behaviour Observed
4	Student using pictures solely for word-solving
13	Student using pictures to predict theme following tutor prompting
13, 21	Student using pictures to predict theme without tutor prompting

Familiarisation of the text

Session 6 I suggested that Alice re-read a text. In *Session 13* Alice suggested I re-read a poem in response to my reading. The latter example is particularly interesting:

While reading a poem I kept stumbling as I read 'there' for 'this' and took no account of the italicised print:

T: There (This) is no place for cows to be, he sh I'll say it again There (this) is no place for cows to be he shouted, and slapped them with seaweed, all the way home.

A: I thought you'd have to read it a few times to know how to shape that bit.

T: To shape that bit yeh.

A: To be able to shape it- it's a different shade of writing (referring to italicised 'This is no place for cows to be').

After I read from the beginning again she recognised the reason for italicisation:

A: It's the cows talking.

T: . . . It's the cows talking cows talking yes that's right so maybe I should have put on a different voice...... 'Cos I haven't read it haven't read it before and you can sort of sense that can't you.

A: Yes.

Table 16.3 summarises these findings.

Table 16.3 Bibliographic knowledge: Familiarisation of the text

Session	Behaviour Observed
6, 7	Student re-read poem following tutor prompting
13, 19	Re-reading suggested by student

Accessing Information

During *Session 9* Alice brought in a poetry book from home. We managed to find a favourite poem by talking about strategies for accessing information such as titles. Alice explained that there was a poem that she wanted to read but she couldn't remember the title. I asked her what it was about. I suggested that we look at the back of the book for titles and first lines. I was able to find it when Alice had told me about it and suggested the beginning letter. In *Session 13* Alice was able to suggest an appropriate place for accessing information:

T: How do you think you could find out if there was a poem about a horse without looking through the pictures?

A: Well in the Contents

T: Yeh.

By *Session 15* I considered her knowledge of ways of accessing information from texts in which the pictures were of some importance. I found that she was not able to use caption text:

T: Where are they from? (referring to picture of ponies. Caption text refers to Shetland ponies)

A: They're from Wales.

T: How can you find out?

A: This bit. (Points to incorrect caption text.)

In *Session 16* she was able to use caption text to find out about a picture:

T: So which of these tells you about that?

A: This one . . .

T: Just read a little bit about this then.

A: Left

T: Yes that tells you it's there . . .

A: Saddles are st still made by hand . . .

During *Session 18* when reading a book about astronomy she also used the caption text with only a little assistance (see Table 16.4).

Table 16.4 Bibliographic knowledge: Accessing information

Session	Behaviour Observed
6, 9	Unable to use Contents to find poem without tutor assistance
13	Student suggested using Contents to access information
15	Unaware of function of caption text
16, 18	Student used caption text to develop knowledge with tutor help

Knowledge about the world

Drawing upon a student's knowledge about the world was certainly motivating. The idea that a student could bring a great deal of knowledge to a text seemed to be a way of empowering the student. The fact that Alice could read words like 'Andromeda' in context suggested that she was able to use specialist knowledge from time to time to read. However, it was difficult to find sufficient examples to show an increase in her control of the learning situation from using knowledge about the world.

Conclusion

This study has demonstrated how a student with reading difficulties increased her control of the reading process over an eight-week period by talking about strategies. The student drew on a wide variety of different types of knowledge to read, the development of which was strongly influenced by the talk of student and tutor. A descriptive system using summary tables was devised which demonstrated the development of the student's reading and the changes in the degree of support given by the tutor. It also analysed student reading within and beyond the level of the word and reading was viewed holistically, a perspective which is not possible when the assessment tool is confined to miscue analysis.

Acknowledgements

This research which forms part of a doctoral thesis was supported by the Economic and Social Research Council. I thank Dr P. Hannon for his useful comments and suggestions in the preparation of this paper.

References

Bryant, P. and Bradley, L. (1985) *Children's Reading Difficulties*. Oxford: Blackwell.

Engelmann, S. and Bruner, E.C. (1983) *Reading Mastery: Distar Reading 1, Presentation Book A*. Chicago: Science Research Associates.

Martin, T. (1989) *The Strugglers*. Milton Keynes: Open University Press.

McNaughton, S. Glynn, T. and Robinson, V. (1987) *Pause, Prompt and Praise*. Birmingham: Positive Products.

Meek, M. (ed.) (1983) *Achieving Literacy*. London: Routledge & Paul.

Mudre, L. and McCormick, S. (1989) Effects of meaning-focused cues on underachieving readers' context use, self-corrections and literal comprehension. *Reading Research Quarterly*, Winter, 89–113.

Rose, T., McEntire, E. and Dowdy, C. (1982) Effects of two error-correction procedures on oral reading. *Learning Disability Quarterly* 5, Spring, 100–105.

17 The Acquisition of English by a Japanese-speaking Child: The Sibilant-sound Attachment as an Influence of Japanese

ASAKO YAMADA-YAMAMOTO

1. Introduction

It is generally said that monolingual English-speaking (E-sp) children do not produce inflectional morphemes, such as the plural and the possessive, in their initial stage of word combinations. The young Japanese-speaking child in the longitudinal case study (Yamada-Yamamoto, 1995a), however, frequently produced what sounded like English inflectional morphemes: he attached a sibilant sound to the end of a word or a group of words from an early stage of word combinations. As the child's English developed, this phenomenon gradually disappeared, although it was still occasionally observed even at a much later time. Based on the analysis, it was concluded that this child's initial sibilant-sound attachment was strongly influenced by the Japanese language which he was learning concurrently with English.

The subject of this case study was my third son called 'Jun'. He came to England when he was 2 years and 1 month old. Jun's exposure to English started when he was 2 years and 2 months. He was regularly exposed to English mainly in the daytime during the week outside the home. At other times, he generally used Japanese at home. The study started when Jun was 3 years and 4 months, covering a period of 1 year and 5 months. It has to be emphasized that during the whole period of data collection,

Jun was involved in active acquisition of Japanese as well as English. Furthermore, in Jun's case, my husband and I gave equal priority to both English and Japanese.

The data were collected frequently on a regular basis each month. They were both video- and audio-recorded, and were later transcribed. For the analysis of Jun's sibilant sound attachments, all the intelligible English utterances with this feature were selected from the monthly samples. Instances of sibilant attachment to Japanese words were also included.

Prior to actual analysis, Jun's mean length of utterance (MLU) was analysed and was compared with the development of MLU of E-sp children studied by Wells (1985). Based on this analysis, it was judged that the developmental profile of Jun's MLU, which was plotted against the length of exposure to English, was nearly comparable to that of the E-sp children, despite the difference in age (see Figure 17.1).

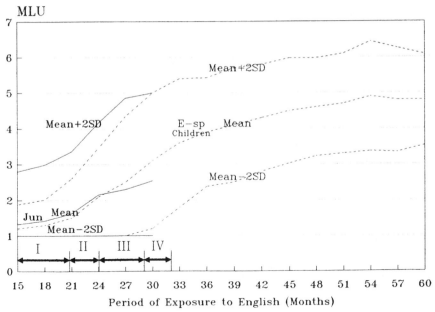

Figure 17.1 Comparison by Exposure Length.

2. Jun's Sibilant-Sound Attachment

Table 17.1 shows examples of Jun's sibilant sound attachment during the data collection period, which was divided into four 'Intervals'. These examples were categorized into three groups: first, those in which the sibilant sound appeared to function as English morphemes; second, those in which the sibilant sound appeared to be used in utterances in a reverse word order to that of English word order; and third, other cases in which the sibilant sound was attached to the places where it was not expected to occur.

In the first 'English-like' category, it is interesting to note that the initial sibilant sound attachment which had appeared to indicate the possessive was dropped in Interval II, and then it was used again in Interval III. Regarding the copula-like sibilant sound attachment, it is noteworthy that in Interval IV, dual use of the copula-like forms was observed in one single utterance. Furthermore, in Interval IV, when the present progressive morpheme began to be produced fairly consistently, he tended to produce utterances in which the real auxiliary was dropped.

Table 17.1 also shows that the second category (i.e. 'Non English-like' category), namely, sibilant attachments in utterances with the reverse word order, gradually disappeared as time passed, but they were still observed even in Interval IV. This is in contrast to those in the third category (i.e. 'Others'), because they were reduced drastically in Interval II.

Table 17.1 Sibilant sound attachment in Jun's utterances

	Interval I (15–19 month)	Interval II (20–23 month)	Interval III (24–28 month)	Interval IV (29–31 month)
English Like	Maskmans belt keys videos twos friend	cf. Jun Mummy cf. Hide chair	cf. big man house Billys birthday	cf.this is spaceship
		this ones mine	my cars change (= My car changes)	hes is my friend mines is broken
	Billys comins	Shins rabbit (= Shin is making a rabbit)	this goes this one	cf. he falling down cf. he making the boat
	Sarahs gone			
Non English Like	bananas eating jellys eating	this ones sleep	this ones same (= The same as this one) this ones pull	this ones fall (= I fell at this place)
		papers reading		
	airplanes noru hit (= People getting on an airplane)			
Others	too manys	lets go Londons	none	none
	black sames			
	look at mes			
	Konnichiwas			

Since in Interval I Jun's sibilant sound attachment occurred frequently and in a diverse fashion, attention should be focused more closely on Interval I and part of Interval II. How his sibilant attachment occurred can be illustrated in Figure 17.2. His sibilant attachment occurred at a sentence medial position in utterances with correct word order, as is shown in Section (1). Jun's sibilant sound attachment also occurred in utterances with incorrect word order, as is shown in Section (2). Jun's

(1)   Utterance Medial Position — English Like

    Ss V: Billys comins (= Billy is coming)
    Ss C: twos friends (= The two people are friends to each other)
            Sarahs gone (= Sarah has gone)
            bins warechatta (= A bottle has got broken)
            botans okkocchatta (= A button has dropped)

      cf. Shins rabbit (= Shin is making a rabbit)
          hes four (= He has got four cards)

      cf. Hides gakkos (= Hide went to school)

    NPs NP: Maskmans belt (= Maskman's belt)
              Wan-Wan Juns friends (= WWJ's friends)
              Hides tama (= Hide's bead)

(2)   Utterance Medial Position — Non English Like

    Os V: bananas eating (= He is eating a banana)
            jellys eating (= I ate jelly)
            this ones hippatte (= Pull this one)
            Mummys koroshita (= I killed my mummy (with a toy sword))

    As V: this ones sleep (= We will sleep on this one)

    As NP: airplanes noru hito (= People getting on an airplane)

(3)   Utterance Final Position — Others

            too manys (= There are many animals)
            this biggers (= This one is bigger)
            all Maskmans (=All are 'Maskman')
     – lets go Londons (= Let's go to London)
     – look at mes (= Look at me)
            no Hides (= Hide did not go)
            Londons (= I went to London)
            this Korakuen Yuenchis (= I saw this at Korakuen Yuenchi)
            childminders (= I went to the childminder's)
            shichiji-s (= It is seven o'clock: shichiji = 7 o'clock)
            yuki-s (= It is snowing: yuki = snow)
            kinono-s (= It is yesterdays)
            hajimeru-s (= Let's start: hajimeru = start)
            Asda Kaimonos (= We will go shopping at Asda: kaimono = shopping)
     + konnichiwa-s (= Hello)
     + Shin-to Hide-s (= Shin and Hide!)

Figure 17.2 Sibilant sound attachment in interval I (or II).

sibilant sound attachment was not only confined to utterances with English vocabulary items; it also occurred with Japanese vocabulary items. Jun's sibilant sound attachment also occurred very frequently in the utterance final position. Examples are shown in Section (3). Examples with exclusively Japanese vocabulary items are also included here.

Two important points can be put forward concerning Jun's sibilant sound attachment. Firstly, it occurred in both single- and multi-word utterances with items of various parts of speech, such as nouns, adjectives, adverbs and verbs, although it occurred most frequently with nouns (see Table 17.2). It was also observed at both utterance-medial and -final positions, although it occurred at the phrasal boundary in all cases. Thus his sibilant sound attachment was represented at the phrasal boundary in a diverse fashion. Secondly, it occurred in utterances which were already well-formed or nearly well-formed in addition to in ill-formed utterances. Instances such as *lets go Londons* and *look at mes* in Section (3) reflect this aspect.

Table 17.2 S-sound attachment to English/Japanese vocabulary

	English Vocabulary	*Japanese Vocabulary*
Noun Phrases	e.g. waters Legos trees	e.g. yuki-s (= Snow)
Verbs	e.g. comins	e.g. shinjatta-s (= Have died)
Adjectives	e.g. sames biggers manys	e.g. okkii-s (= Big)
Adverbs	e.g. heres	
Others	e.g. nos	e.g. konnichiwa-s (= Hello)

Judging from the first point, namely, sibilant sound attachment in a diverse fashion, it seemed that this phenomenon could be regarded as an indication of the influence of the Japanese bound morphemes which actually have diverse grammatical as well as semantic functions (Kuno, 1973; T. Okubo, 1977 and Yamada-Yamamoto, 1995a). Concerning the second point, namely sibilant sound attachment even to already well-formed in addition to ill-formed English sentences, it seemed that Jun's sibilant attachment was an indication of his attempt to make his utterances sound more English.

3. Interpretation of Jun's Sibilant Attachment Phenomenon

Indication of English structure

Superficially, some of Jun's initial sibilant sound attachment seem to reflect English inflectional morphemes, namely, plural, the third person singular present tense of the verb, and the possessive. The English-like category in Table 17.1 includes some such instances in Interval I, as have already been mentioned. None of these possibilities, however, were supported, either, due to lack of consistency in the way Jun used the sibilant sound and the actual meaning, or due to a clear lack of evidence to support the suggestion. Firstly, his sibilant sound did not seem to be related to the English singular versus plural dichotomy. For example, he said *keys* referring to only one key. He said *videos* and *televisions,* as he was pointing at a video camera and a television set. Secondly, there are too few instances of the sibilant attachment which appeared to be the third person singular present tense of the verb. Since there are only four such cases during the whole data-collection period, it was judged that this suggestion was not supported. Thirdly, Jun's early speech includes relatively frequent instances where the sibilant sound seemed to indicate the English possessive morpheme. He said *Maskmans belt*, for example. Developmentally, however, the number of such instances suddenly decreased later. In Interval II, he almost always omitted the possessive morpheme. Jun insisted on producing the incorrect form *Jun mummy* rather than the correct form of `Jun's mummy' in the conversation. Around this time, he may have hypothesized that zero morpheme usage should be used to indicate possession. If the sibilant sound had been used as an English possessive marker from the beginning, there would not have been any reason for him to dismiss it, especially as his knowledge of English was greater in the later period. The fact that he dropped the sibilant sound might well be good evidence that the original usage of the sibilant sound was not recognized as the English possessive morpheme.

The possibility that Jun's sibilant sound reflects the English contracted copula or auxiliary was also ruled out. Towards the end of the data-collection period, that is, Interval IV, Jun produced many utterances with the uncontracted form, namely, `is' in Subject-Complement type utterances. Table 17.1 includes one such utterance: *this is spaceship*. During the same period, however, he also produced utterances with dual use of copula-like forms such as *hes is my friend* and *mines is broken*, as mentioned previously. In these 'dual use' instances, the sibilant attachment of the subject NP was always pronounced very quickly as if it formed a unit with the Noun Phrase. In addition, the second uncontracted form, namely 'is', tended to be produced showing a stress. If the sibilant sound had already had the status of a real copula, there would have been no dual use of copulas. Based on such an observation, it was judged that the sibilant sound initially produced did not reflect the English copula. Further, as was also mentioned earlier, when Jun began to produce the present progressive morpheme fairly consistently in Interval IV, he tended to omit the auxiliary, whether or not it was contracted, as is shown in the examples *he falling down* and *he making the boat*. If the initial sibilant sound had had the status of auxiliary, it would not have been dropped when he started to produce the present progressive form. Based on these observations, it was judged that the initial sibilant sound attachment did not have the status of either an English copula or auxiliary.

Influence of Japanese structure

Pursuing the hypothesis of the influence of the features of Japanese, an error analysis was conducted. If the instances of the sibilant sound attachments had actually been influenced by the Japanese structure, then we can predict that certain cases would result in error and the other cases would result in non-error, from the viewpoint of the English structure. If such a prediction turns out to be true, we can judge that the Japanese influence hypothesis can be supported. In other words, the error analysis indicates that when the structures of the two languages were similar, the replacement of the Japanese particle by the sibilant sound in a Japanese utterance, together with the replacement of Japanese vocabulary by the English equivalent, would have resulted in correctly structured English, and when the structures were different, the replacement would have resulted in incorrectly structured English.

English and Japanese have similar structures in the following limited cases as is shown in Table 17.3. The first one is the Subject–Complement type sentence in English with the subject being the third person singular. For this type of sentence, the sequence of 'the Subject, the sibilant sound and the Complement' in English looks similar to the Japanese structure of 'the Subject, subject-marking particle -*ga*, and the Complement'. The second one is the genitive construction in English. For this type of construction, the sequence of 'the Noun Phrase indicating the possessor, the sibilant sound and the Noun Phrase indicating the possessed' resembles the Japanese genitive construction of 'the Noun indicating the possessor, the possessive-marking particle -*no*, and the Noun indicating the possessed'. In these two cases, the replacement of the particle by the sibilant sound would have resulted in the production of correct English structures. On other occasions, however, the replacement of the particles by the sibilant sound and the translation of vocabulary from Japanese to English would have resulted in incorrect English structures.

Table 17.3 Structural similarities and differences between English and Japanese in relation to Jun's medial position sibilant sound attachment

Function of S-attachment	Relevant Structures English	Japanese	Similar or Different	Error in English
Subject-marking (SC-type, 3rd person singular present)	S-'s C	S-ga C	similar	No Error
Possessive-marking	NP's NP	NP-no NP	similar	No Error
Subject-marking (other SC-type and LV-containing)	S Cop C S V	S-ga C S-ga V	different	Error
Object-marking	V O	O-o V	different	Error
Locative-marking (A realized as NP)	V A	A-ni V	different	Error
Enumeration	NP and NP	Np-to NP-to	different	Error
Comparison	Adj prep NP	NP-to Adj	different	Error

It was found that these predictions concerning correctness or incorrectness would explain almost all the examples with the 'medial-position' sibilant attachment. Due to such an ability to predict errors, it was concluded that the interpretation, assuming the influence of the Japanese particle, should be supported, at least for the sibilant attachment which occurred in a medial position in the utterance.

Additional evidence for this Japanese particle hypothesis is also found in Jun's production of all the combinations of English NP with the sibilant sound, Japanese NP with the sibilant sound, English NP with the particle, and Japanese NP with the particle. This shows that the replacement of the Japanese particle with the sibilant sound or the replacement of the sibilant sound with the Japanese particle took place with both English and Japanese NPs (see Table 17.4).

Table 17.4 English/Japanese NP and S-sound/particle combinations

Combinations	Examples
(1) English NP + S-sound	e.g. twos friend
(2) Japanese NP + S-sound	e.g. botans okkochatta. (= A button has dropped)
(3) English NP + Japanese Particle	e.g. you-no ban (= your turn)
(4) Japanese NP + Japanese Particle	e.g. Onna-no happybirthdays (= A girl's birthday party)

A separate analysis was conducted during the period of Interval I, concerning Jun's use of Japanese particles in Japanese. It was revealed that at this time not only did he use the Japanese particles in a diverse fashion but also his use of the Japanese particles was comparable to that of Japanese children learning Japanese in Japan (e.g. A. Okubo, 1967 and Clancy, 1985). It is quite reasonable to suppose, therefore, that Jun transferred the features of Japanese to his acquisition of English.

It was thus confirmed that the hypothesis assuming the influence of the Japanese particles should be supported concerning Jun's initial sibilant sound attachment. At the same time, it was found that a much broader interpretation, which assumes an influence from the use of the Japanese bound morphemes in general, could explain more instances of Jun's sibilant attachment, since the concept of bound morpheme is wider as it includes both particles and auxiliaries. Since Japanese utterance-final particles and Japanese auxiliaries share certain characteristics, both from formal and meaning points of view (T. Okubo, 1977; see also Figures 17.4 and 17.5 in the Appendix), many instances of `final-position' sibilant attachment can actually be interpreted as either an indication of influence from the use of Japanese utterance-final particles or as an indication of a Japanese auxiliary or a combination of both.

Furthermore, since Japanese bound morphemes are used only at the constituent boundary to make up a sense unit, Jun's tendency to attach the sibilant sound to the end of utterances, can be interpreted as an indication of his attempt to form a phrasal unit or a sense unit (cf. Tanaka, 1981). In other words, by attaching the sibilant sound to a word or words, he subconsciously made it a unit corresponding to the Japanese sense unit, as the sibilant sound functions as if it were a bound morpheme. The fact that he produced only one or two words, which appear to correspond to the beginning of the plausible Japanese utterances, could be interpreted as his attempt at minimal communication when he had something to say, but he could not express it because of his lack of English. For example, he said *Londons* meaning 'I went to London', interpreted from the context. He did not say any more than that because he did not know the English syntax to express the Japanese equivalent.

English flavour

As we have seen so far, most of the instances of sibilant attachment can be explained by the influence of a wider concept of Japanese bound morphemes in general. However, there are still some instances which cannot be explained even by this broader bound morpheme hypothesis. It should be pointed out that Jun's sibilant sound attachment occurred in an utterance where it was not expected, following Jun's observed use of the bound morphemes in Japanese. The sibilant attachment of this category is shown in the examples with the plus mark (+) in Figure 17.2. He said *konnichiwa-s*, meaning 'hello'. He also said *Shin-to Hide-s*, addressing his brothers. It is likely that this indicates his attempt to make his utterances sound `English'. The sibilant attachment also occurred in English utterances which had already been well-formed or nearly well-formed. For example, he said *lets go Londons* and *look at mes* (see examples with the minus mark (–) in Figure 17.2). Jun's sibilant attachment in these cases can be interpreted as indicating that he may have over-extended his application of the `English-flavour' sibilant attachment unnecessarily.

Such an interpretation is based on the fact that English constituent boundaries often coincide with sibilant sound attachment exemplified by the morphemes such as the plural, and the possessive, or certain verb forms, or the contracted copula and the auxiliaries. Because of such an incidental feature of the English constituent boundaries, Jun may have assumed that English constituents tend to end with the sibilant sound. From the observation of the running discourse of English spoken around him, Jun might have formed the impression that English often contained the sibilant sound at an utterance boundary.

4. Summary

In summary, the above explanation interprets Jun's sibilant attachment phenomenon as having occurred as a combined effect of his observation of English and his knowledge of Japanese. This explanation means that the `English flavour' hypothesis and the hypothesis assuming an influence of Japanese structures are not mutually exclusive. On the contrary, they are complementary (see Figure 17.3 for a schematic representation).

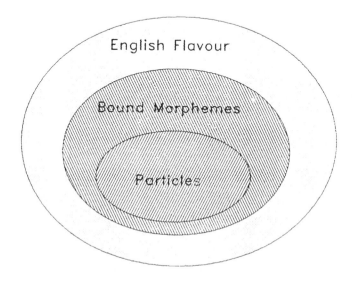

Figure 17.3 Sibilant-sound attachment in Jun's utterances.

Developmentally, utterance-final sibilant sound attachment, which can be interpreted as being used as an `English flavour' and as having been influenced by the general use of Japanese bound morphemes, radically decreased in Interval II. Medial-position sibilant attachments gradually disappeared, although those with incorrect word order were occasionally observed even at the end of the data collection period. Separate analyses suggested that English Verb+Object word order was acquired probably between the end of Interval I and the beginning of Interval II (Yamada-Yamamoto, 1993), and that the word orders Verb + Adverb and Preposition + NP were acquired at some time during Interval III (Yamada-Yamamoto, 1995b). The fact that sibilant attachment with incorrect word order occurred, even after the correct word orders were acquired, could be an indication that the Japanese syntactic devices were automatically adopted by Jun as a default. Since his knowledge of Japanese syntax was more deeply rooted, it was sometimes present even after major English structures were acquired.

Appendix

---

(1) Utterance Medial Position

Role (or case) Particle
   e.g.   Watashi-*ga* John-*to* machi-*ni* ikimasu.
          (= I am going to town with John)

Focus Particle
   e.g.   John-ga tegami-o kaki-masu. Mary-*mo* kaki-masu.
          (= John writes a letter. So does Mary.)

Conjunctive Particle
   e.g.   Onaka-ga-suita-*kara* gohan-o tabe-mashita.
          (= As I was hungry, I had a meal.)

(2) Utterance Final Position

Utterance Final Particle
   e.g.   Heya-o soji-shi-mashita-*ka*?
          (= Did you clean the room?)

   e.g.   Kondo omocha katte-*ne*.
          (= Buy me a toy next time, please.)

Figure 17.4 Japanese particles

(1) Auxiliary
      e.g. Taro-wa gakusei-*da*.
            (= Taro is a student.)

(2) Auxiliaries agglutinated sequentially
      e.g. Taro-wa tabako-o kai-ni-ika *-se-rare-na-katta-yooda-sooda*.
            (= Taro is reported to be likely not to have been made to go
            to buy cigarettes.)

(3) Similarity between Particles and Auxiliaries
      e.g. Taro-wa chiisai-*yo*.
            (= Taro is small <particle>)
      e.g. Taro-wa chiisai-*desu*.
            (= Taro is small <auxiliary>)

      e.g. Taro-wa gakusei-*yo*.
            (= Taro is a student <affirmative particle>)
      e.g. Taro-wa gakusei-*da-yo*.
            (= Taro is a student <affirmative auxiliary and particle>)

Figure 17.5 Japanese bound morphemes.

References.

Clancy, P. M. (1985) The acquisition of Japanese. In D.I. Slobin (ed.) *The Crosslinguistic Study of Language Acquisition. Volume 1: The Data*. Hillsdale, NJ: Lawrence Erlbaum Associates. 373–524.

Kuno, S. (1973) *The Structure of the Japanese Language*. Cambridge, MA: The MIT Press.

Okubo, A. (1967) *Yoji no Gengo Hattatsu* (Language Development in Young Children; in Japanese). Tokyo: Tokyo-do.

Okubo, T. (1977) *Shin Nihon Bunpo Nyumon* (An Introduction to New Japanese Grammar; in Japanese). Tokyo: Sanseido.

Tanaka, M. (1981) Structural development of the simple sentence in Japanese children. In P.S. Dale and D. Ingram (eds) *Child Language — An International Perspective* (pp.59–72). Baltimore: University Park Press.

Wells, G. (1985) *Language Development in the Pre-school Years*. Cambridge: Cambridge University Press.

Yamada-Yamamoto, A. (1993) The acquisition of English syntax by a Japanese-speaking child: with special emphasis on the VO-sequence acquisition *Proceedings of Child Language Seminar* (pp.109–19). University Plymouth.

— (1995a) *The Acquisition of English Syntax by A Japanese-speaking Child: From Left Branching to Right Branching*. Tokyo: Liber Press.

— (1995b) The acquisition of English by a Japanese-speaking child: with special emphasis on the acquisition of the VA sequence and the prepositional phrase, *Proceedings of the 6th Conference on Second Language Research in Japan* (pp.1–20). International University of Japan.